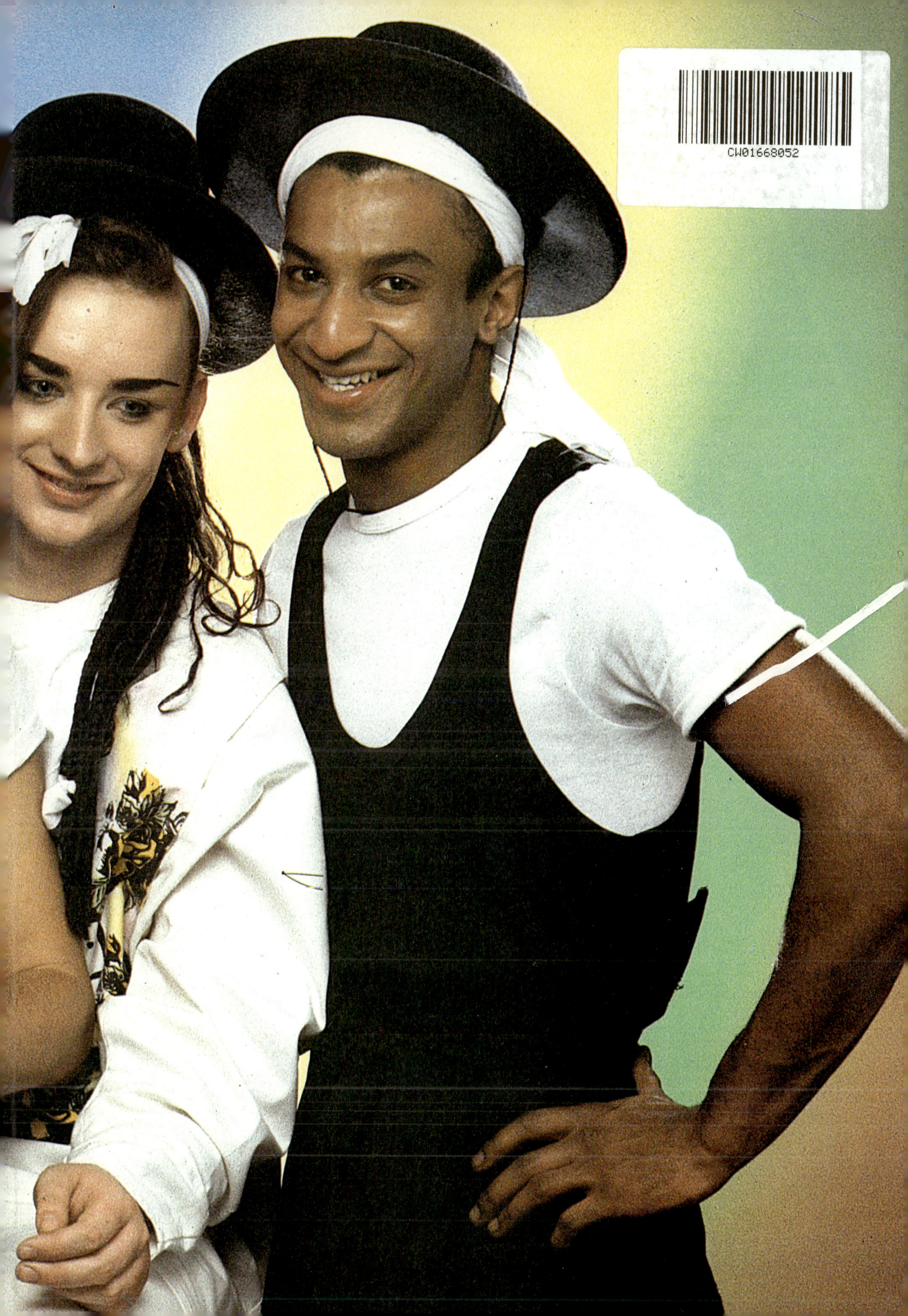

CW01668052

This book was devised and produced by
Multimedia Publications (UK) Ltd

Editor: Richard Rosenfeld
Production: Arnon Orbach
Design: John Strange
Picture Research: Helena Beaufoy

Copyright © Multimedia Publications
(UK) Ltd 1984

First published 1984 by
The Hamlyn Publishing Group Limited
London · New York · Sydney · Toronto
Astronaut House, Feltham, Middlesex,
England.

All rights reserved. No part of this publication may be reproduced, stored in a retrieval system, or transmitted, in any form or by any means, electronic, mechanical, photocopying, recording or otherwise, without the permission of The Hamlyn Publishing Group Limited and the copyright holder(s).

Origination by D. S. Colour International
Ltd, London. Printed in Spain by Cayfosa,
Barcelona
Dep. Leg. B-28946 - 1984

BOY GEORGE
Fashion & Make-up Book

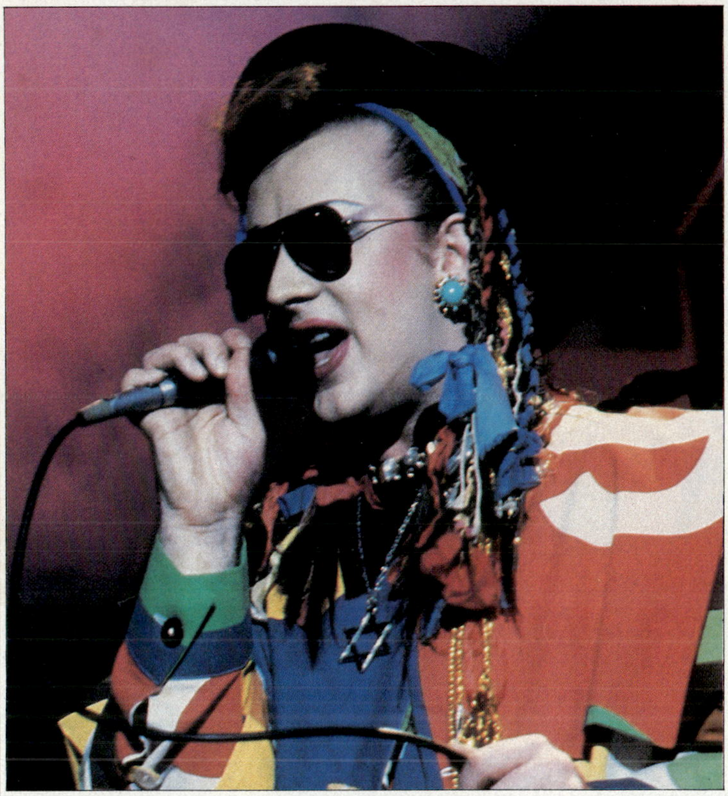

Wayne and Gerardine Winder, Christina Saunders

BOY GEORGE
Fashion & Make-up Book

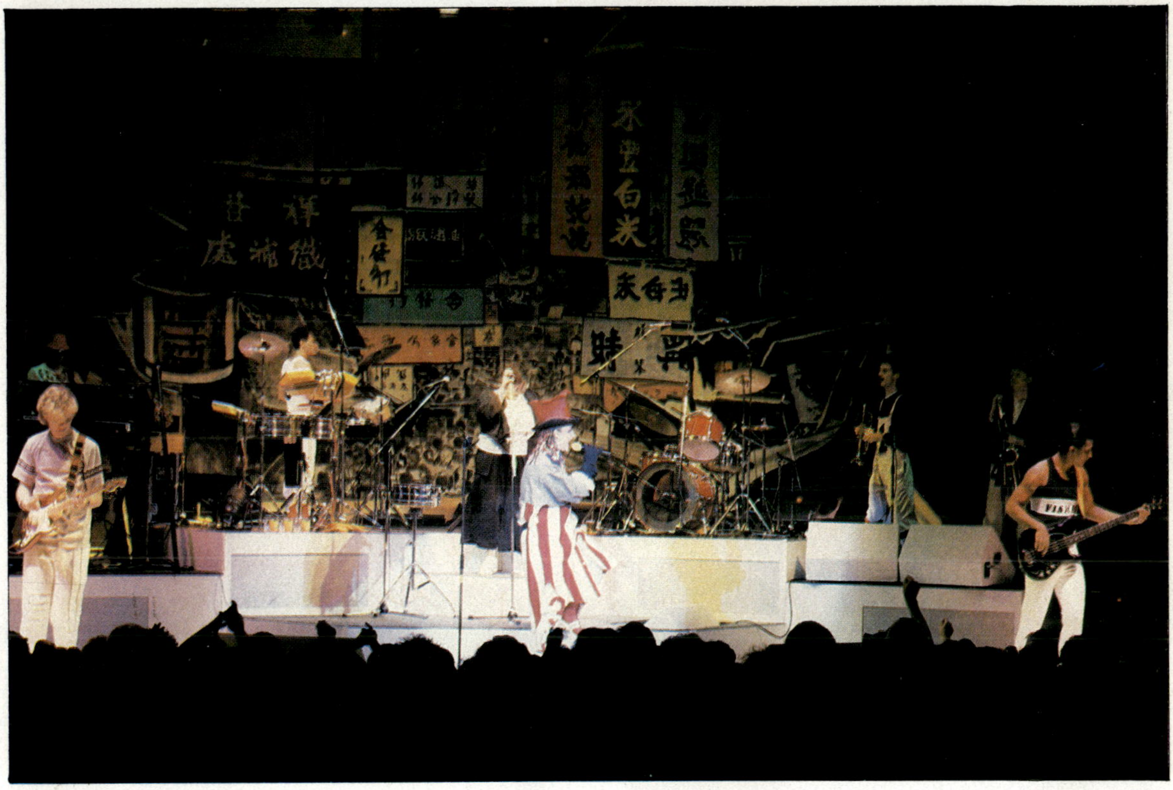

Hamlyn
London · New York · Sydney · Toronto

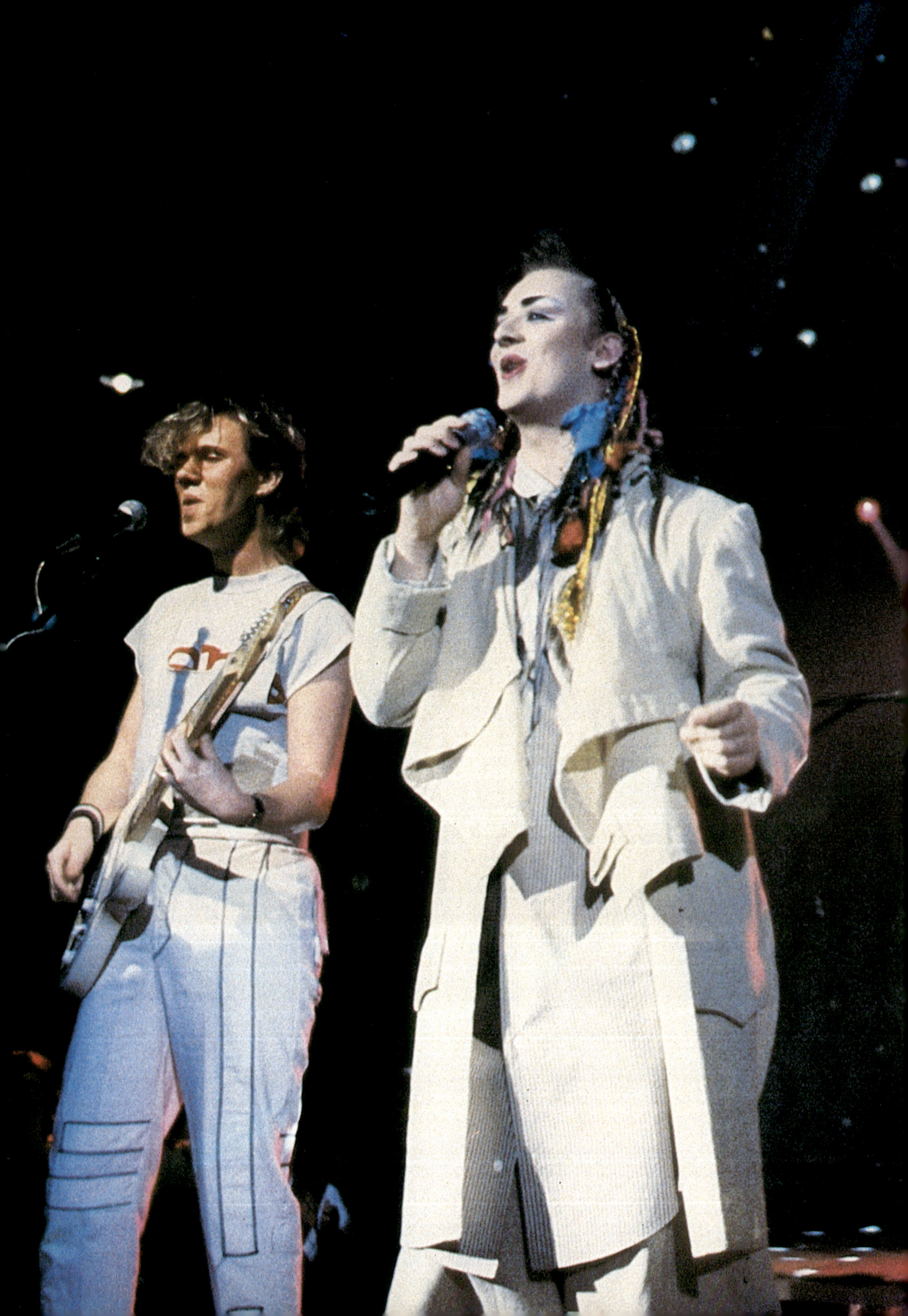

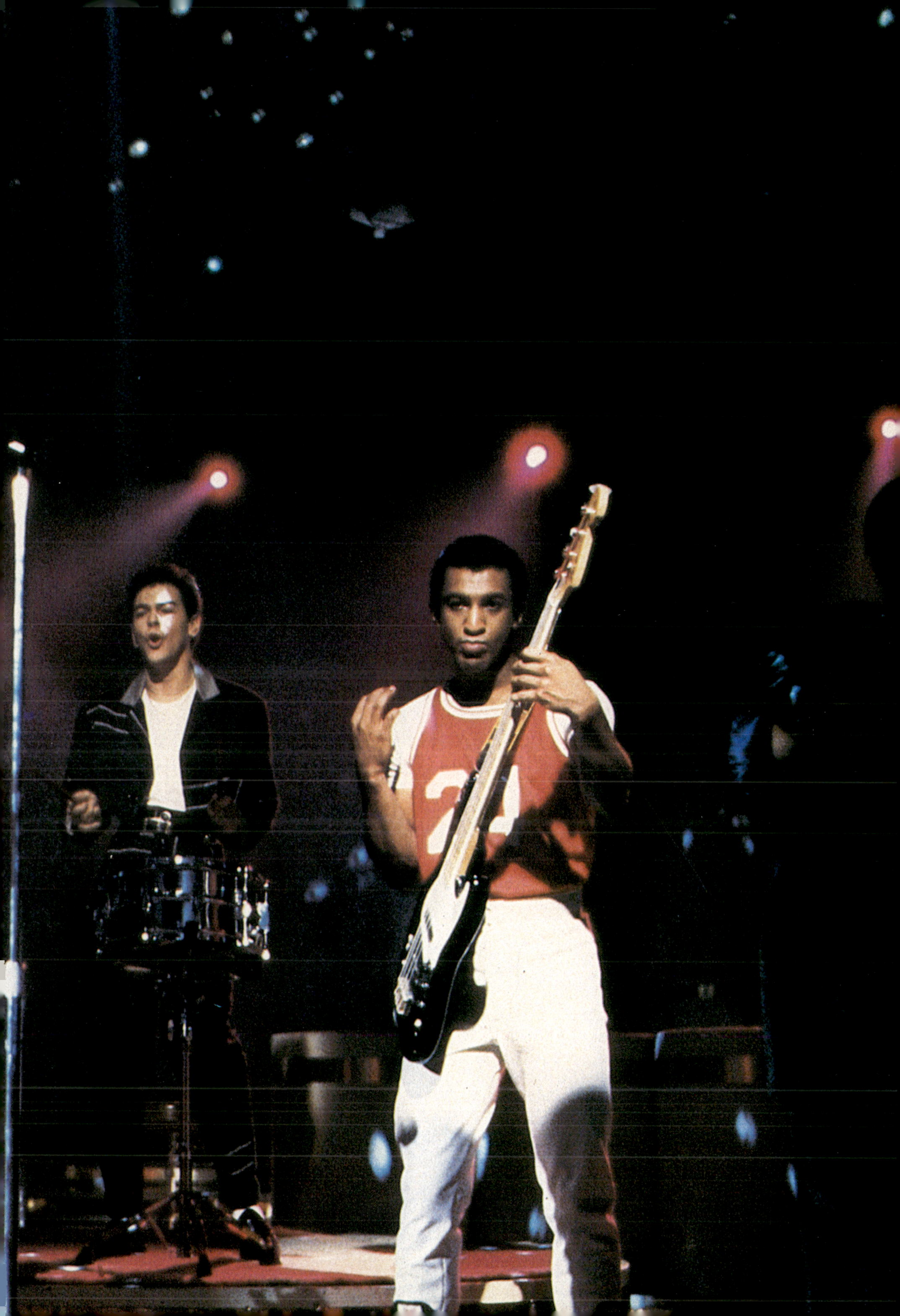

Introduction

Boy George is the most alarming, outrageous and original dresser to hit the pop scene in the past 10 years. His riotously inspired image has grabbed the newspaper headlines and the public imagination as much as any of Culture Club's smash hits.

After the boring jeans and T-shirts of most rock 'n' roll bands, or the harsh horrors of the punk era, Boy George has developed an exciting look with his clothes and make-up which is at once warm, colorful and friendly as well as bizarre, shocking and exotic.

And his fabulously flamboyant fashion has given the rag trade its biggest boost since David Bowie first pranced onto the stage dressed as Ziggy Stardust. Fashion magazines are falling over themselves to dress their top models as Boy George.

Gloriously dressed

The Boy George fashion craze is big business. But you don't need to be a millionaire to dress like Boy George. After all, the star himself was penniless when he first appeared gloriously dressed on the London nightclub scene in the early eighties. Unlike the expensive young executive chic of Duran Duran, all you need to copy Boy George is a little imagination to combine caftans with straw hats and vivid eye make-up.

The look is deliberately sexually ambiguous – just like Boy George himself. It looks as good on girls as it does on boys.

Although his style has sharpened up these days into superstar glamor and he has his own designer to work with him and develop his themes, the real secret of Boy George's stunning appearance is his ability to pick up fresh ideas and then to blend them with existing ones.

Being a seasoned world traveller, Boy George adapts garments from the Japanese kimono to the American flag. He sends home

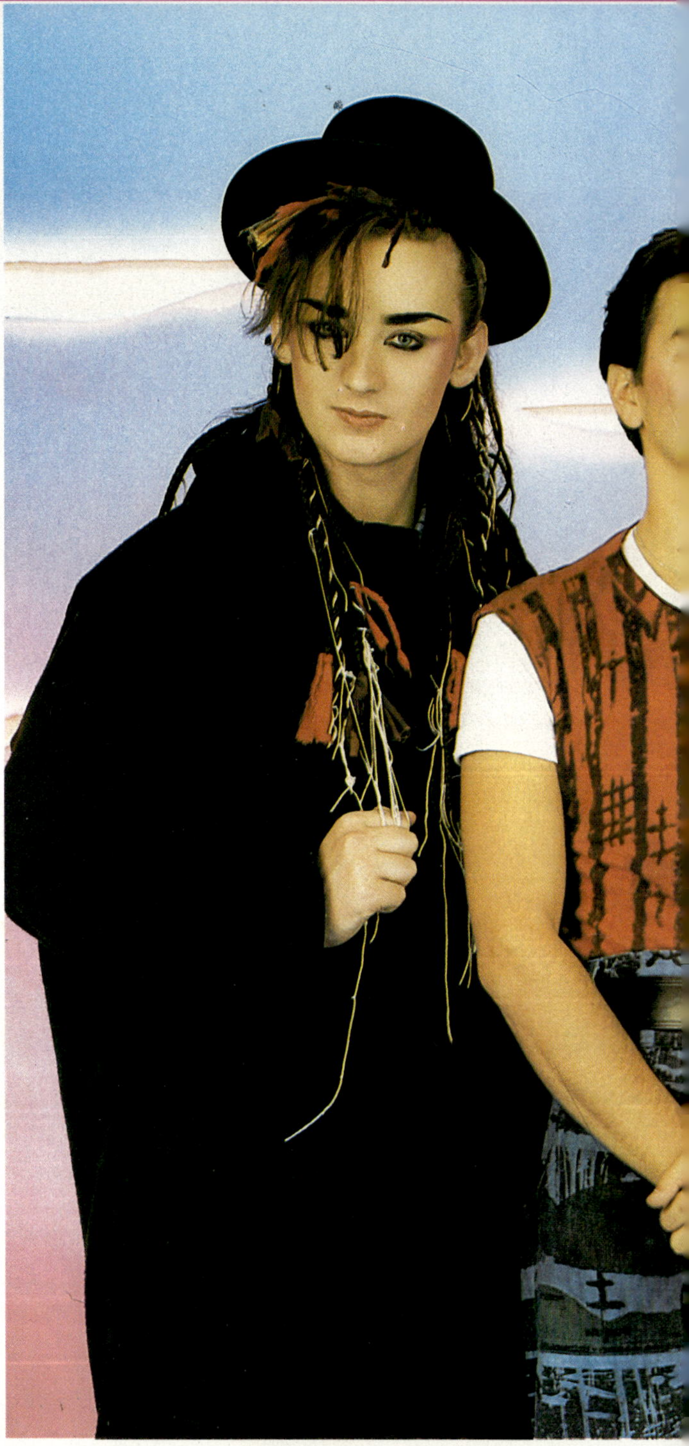

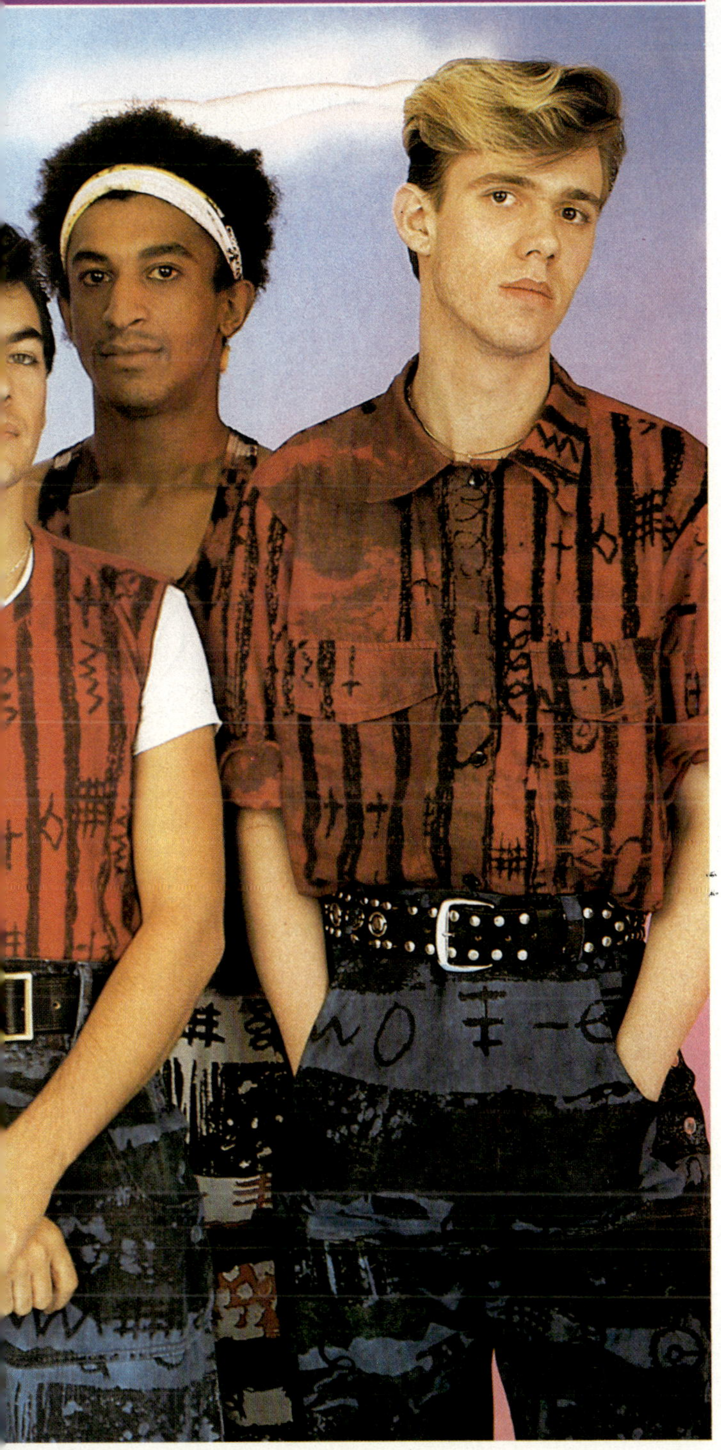

hundreds of postcards to his designer from wherever he is visiting with ideas for new outfits.

Even before George hit the big-time, he was plundering the rag bag of fashion, always coming up with something breathtakingly brilliant.

Where it all began

The schoolboy streak of rebellion – George was always in trouble for his clothes and dyeing his hair bright orange – flowered in the nightclubs of London and Birmingham, England, in the late seventies and early eighties. The new romantic posers, repelled by the violence of the punks, flocked together for support.

Not surprisingly, George was the most photographed face on the scene. After going through the Bowie, punk and rockabilly phases, he developed his own style. Amazingly, despite all the glitter, jewellery, make-up and finery, George was dressing from thrift shops and second-hand stores. At about the age of 17 he realized that you don't need to be wealthy to be glamorous and stylish.

George became a minor celebrity on the nightclub scene where life was one endless party. He experimented with every style – Rocky Horror, Hollywood stars, even nuns – and soon outstripped the most outrageous opposition.

World conqueror

But this was not enough. He set out to shock and ended up conquering the whole world and converting millions to his dashing point of view.

The distinctive Culture Club style emerged when George worked with a designer in a London shop and together they developed the Star of David T-shirts and the exotic symbolism of hobos and rastafarians.

As Culture Club became more than mere singing mannequins, Boy George's look became more sophisticated. He grew his hair like Rita Hayworth, employed a make-up artist and appeared in ever more fascinating patterns and prints.

But Boy George does not believe in dressing up just to impress people or in wasting a lot of money trying to look like a star. He still finds new and cheap things all around him and never tires of looking for new ideas in old clothes. That is the secret of the Boy George style. And anyone can do it.

FASHION TIPS

All the clothes featured in this book are easy to make. None of them have darts or any tailored shaping; there is a minimum of curved seams, and for the most part the shapes are those of the basic ethnic clothes, such as caftans, which women have been cutting and sewing, without any training in dressmaking and without any patterns to help them, for centuries.

Sleeves are full and generally made to be worn pushed up, so a few centimetres more or less here, or on the side seams, are not going to ruin the shape of the garment. Provided the guidelines given below are followed, there is no reason why even a completely inexperienced dressmaker should not be able to make highly successful garments from the patterns given here.

Making the patterns
Always make your pattern before buying the fabric, as this will save you from buying too much and thereby wasting money.

Finding paper large enough to make the pattern can be a problem. You may have to stick several large pieces of paper together (tissue paper or large sheets of used wrapping paper can be very useful – iron them before using them, though, so that there are no misleading wrinkles). Dressmaker's pattern paper, with large squares already ruled on it, can be bought in fabric shops but it is very expensive and the shapes of the patterns in this book are so straightforward, being based for the most part on right angles and squared-off shapes, that it would really be a waste of money to buy it.

You could also draw your patterns on sheets of newspaper, but be sure that they are at least one month old, preferably more, so that the print has dried out completely and cannot mark your fabric.

In addition to large sheets of paper you will also need:

- An ordinary ruler and also, if possible, a long metre rule for drawing long lines accurately.
- A set square – absolutely essential for making and checking right-angles, otherwise you might end up with seams which are slightly twisted.
- A tape measure – make sure that it is fairly new, not an old stretched one, and marked in centimetres.
- Graph paper – you will find that it is helpful to make a small sketch to scale, with your measurements written on it, to guide you when making the full-size pattern pieces.
- A pencil and felt-tip (to be used to draw up the pattern and make marks on it).

You can cut out with a minimum of pattern pieces – for example, with one front pattern, flipping it over to make the other side or laying it on doubled fabric – but it is much better to make a complete pattern, with two fronts, two sleeves and so on as this makes it easier to work out an economical layout, saving fabric and therefore money.

The cut out

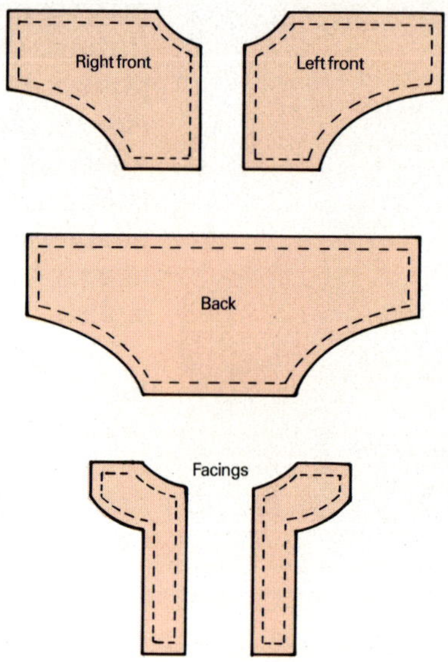

Checking
When you have drawn up one of each pattern piece (one sleeve, one front, a back and so on), check them. Check that all the right angles are accurate and that side and shoulder seams will match – it is much easier to correct mistakes on the pattern than on the finished garment. In order to check, it helps to draw in the sewing line, as opposed to the cutting line, and to measure this rather than the cutting line.

When you are satisfied, cut along the cutting line of the pattern pieces then use them to make further pieces (the other sleeve, the other front) as they are required.

When you have made all your pattern pieces, mark them – right front, left front and so on – and make a further check that seams match. Label the side which will be uppermost when it is placed on the fabric and make sure that you have matching pairs, not identical pieces, where necessary: nothing is more annoying than cutting up an expensive fabric only to find that you have two left fronts instead of a left and a right, but it is unfortunately all too easily done!

It also helps to read the description of how to make up the garment and check that you understand how it fits together. If you are in any doubt as to whether you have got it right, draw a mini-version of each pattern piece and pin them together to see if your conception of the pattern works.

Trial mini trouser pattern

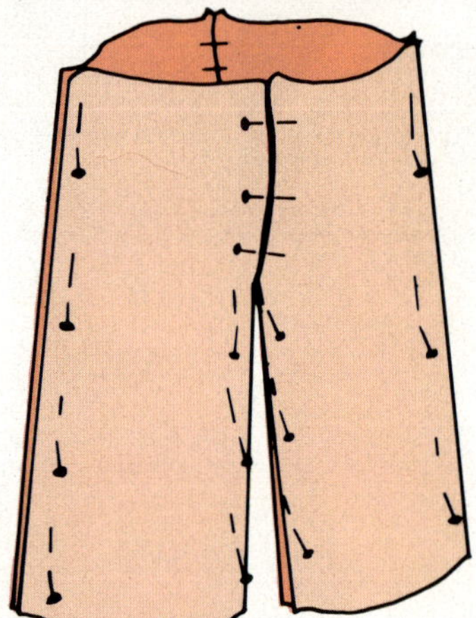

Buying the fabric
Before buying the fabric, work out exactly how much you need by laying out the pattern pieces and juggling round with them to achieve an economical lay-out.

In most of these patterns the back and sleeves are cut all in one, so you will need a wide (150cm/60in) fabric unless you alter the pattern (*see instructions opposite*).

Most shops will be willing to help if you take pattern pieces with you to check how much fabric you will need. If you are thinking of using a patterned fabric (for example a tartan pattern for the jacket on *page 26*) you must add on extra to ensure that you can match up the pattern across the front and at the side seams and sleeves. If you are planning to use an absolutely plain fabric, however, you can work out how much you will need at home.

Clear a space on the floor and mark off the proposed width of your fabric (you can use things like a join in the carpet, your tape measure or a metre rule as guides), then lay out your pattern pieces and move them

The pattern pieces
(a) with nap

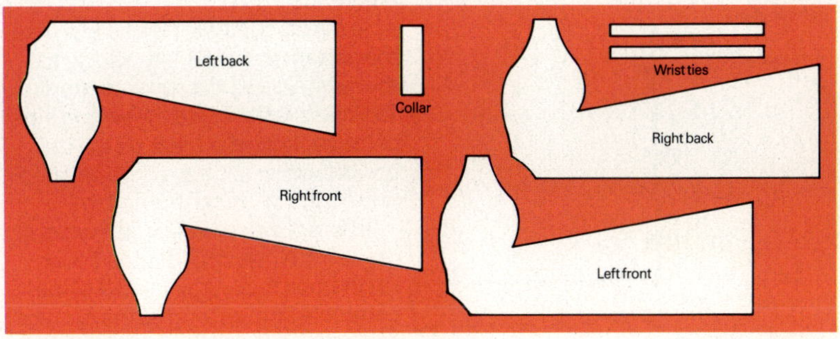

(b) without nap

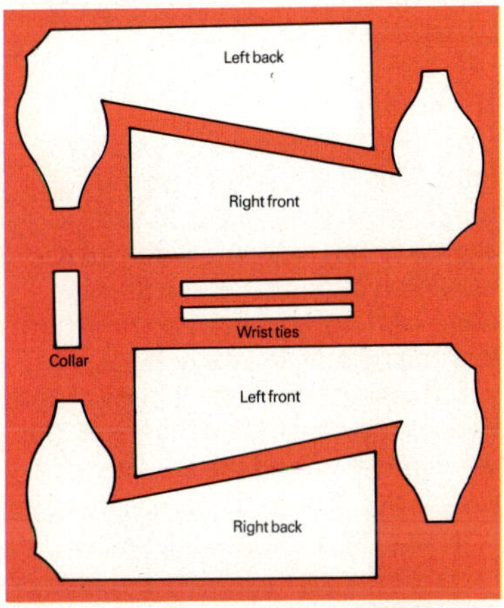

around until you have achieved a satisfactory layout. You may find that you could use 120cm/45in-wide fabric, or 150cm/60in-wide, using a different layout.

If you are intending to choose a fabric which has a nap (like velvet, where the pile should stroke downwards when worn) you will need to place all the pattern pieces lying in one direction, but if there is no nap you can jigsaw them together.

However, all fabric has a 'grain', which is particularly important in heavier material. If you look closely at a piece of uncut fabric, you will see that the grain runs parallel to the line of the uncut edge. Try to keep your larger pattern pieces lying straight down the grain – if you were to cut out a back down the grain and a front across the grain you would find that however carefully you joined them they would not hang well.

Altering the pattern

If you see a fabric which you very much like but find that it is not wide enough, it may be possible to make a simple alteration to the pattern so that you can use it. Many of the patterns given here have the sleeve cut in one with the main body, but in some cases (the tailcoat, the tartan jacket and the wrap-over jacket) you could easily separate off the sleeve pattern by continuing the line from the side seam up to the shoulder (*see diagram below*). Cut along this line and then add seam allowances (1.5cm/⅝in) along each edge.

The sleeve will still be in two sections, a front and a back, with a seam down from the shoulder to the wrist as well as an under-arm seam. To eliminate this (now unnecessary) seam, just cut off the seam allowance (if one has been included) and lay this top sleeve line on a fold in the fabric, to cut one full sleeve.

Attached and separated sleeves

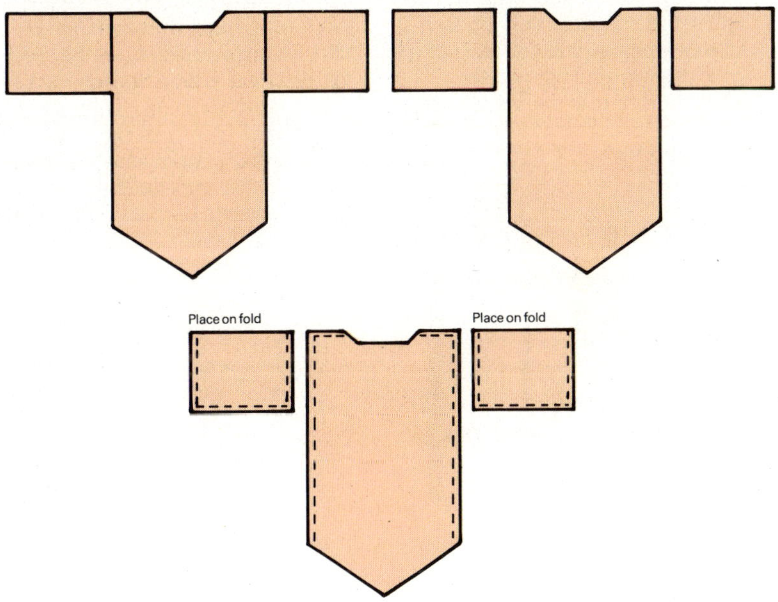

Cutting out

Accurate cutting out is very important if you want your clothes to look good – if the cut edge is crooked then the seam will tend to be crooked as well, so the finished garment will not hang well.

Lay all the pattern pieces on the fabric in their correct positions and put weights on top to hold them in position. You can buy dressmaker's weights – which are like heavy counters – at haberdashery shops, but you can also use other small, not too heavy objects to the same effect.

Using tailor's chalk (also from haberdashery shops or counters), draw round each pattern piece, then remove the pattern and the weights and cut out the fabric. You can pin the pattern to the fabric and cut along the edge, but you will find it far easier to cut straight lines and accurate curves using the tailor's chalk method.

Make sure that you have very sharp fabric shears – beg, borrow or steal them if necessary!

If you are using a patterned fabric, for example when making the tartan jacket, choose a dominant feature such as a red line, and mark the point where this occurs on your pattern (*see diagram*) so that you can use it to check that you cut both fronts, sleeves etcetera at the same level.

Using a tartan fabric

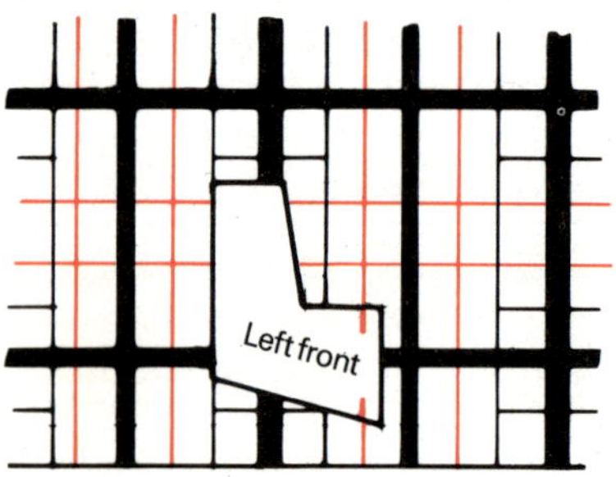

Pinning or tacking

You can tack seams before stitching them but it is often a lot quicker, and every bit as good, if not better, simply to pin them. Most machines will run over the pins without any difficulty and if you do – very occasionally – have to replace a broken needle it is still a lot less trouble than laboriously tacking every seam and then unpicking the tacking stitches (not always easy) when the seam has been stitched.

Place the pins at right angles to the cut edge so that the presser foot can easily run over them. If you have never used this method before, practise on a spare piece of fabric: you will soon get used to it and after that you will rarely need to bother with tacking.

Pinning at right angles

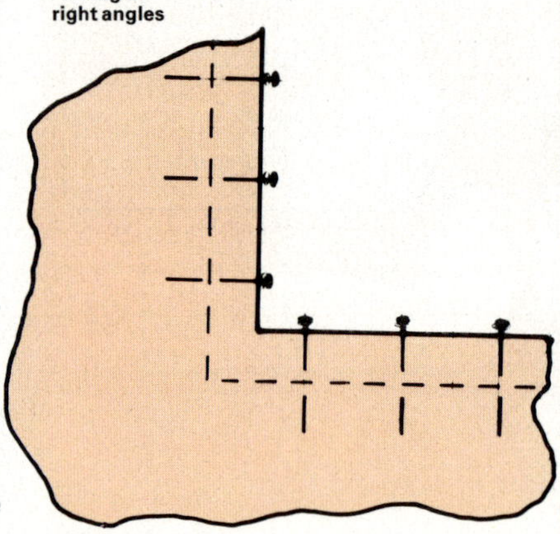

Sewing a seam

Straight seams are very important if the finished garment is to hang right, so if you are not used to sewing or if you are using an unfamiliar machine it is a good idea to practise. Get the stitch length right – too long and the stitches will show, too short and they will tend to make the seam rather stiff. Do not sew slowly, as the seam will just tend to wobble, but practise sewing in short sharp bursts. It is a good idea to put masking tape on the base plate of your machine, 1.5cm/⅝in away from the needle hole, as a guide to help to keep an even seam.

Keeping the seam straight

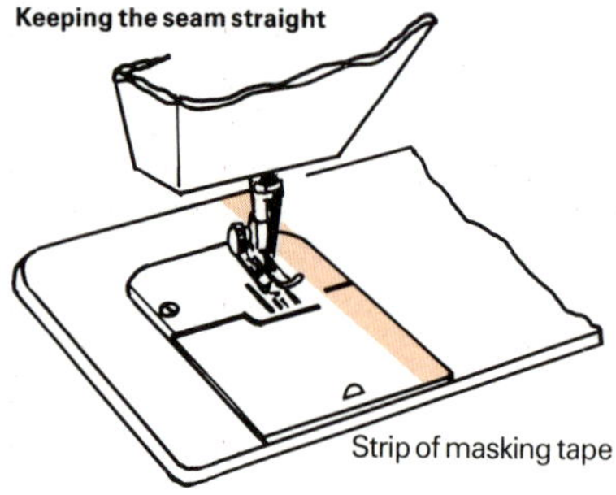

Interfacings

Apart from the interfacing of the jerkin (*page 15*), none of the patterns given here include interfacings, but if you want to give a professional-looking finish to collars and cuffs it would be a good idea to add one to the shirt.

Iron-on interfacing tends to wrinkle the material after a few washes, so it is best to use the sew-in kind. Do not buy a very stiff interfacing as this will make the collar look starchy and unnatural. If you use a light-weight cotton for the shirt you can use the same fabric for the interfacing, provided that the pattern does not show through. Otherwise, use a woven cotton interfacing for the collar and cuffs of the shirt and the collar of the sportsman's nightshirt and a slightly heavier one for the ethnic coat.

To interface a two-piece collar, use the pattern to cut the interfacing to the same size as the collar sections. Tack the interfacing to the wrong side of the section which will be the top (visible) collar section of the finished garment, then make the collar.

To interface a collar or cuff which is made from one strip doubled over, cut the interfacing to one half of the pattern (a strip as long as the pattern and half the width). Tack it to the side which will be the outer side, then make a few catch-stitches down the inner long edge. Finish making the collar or cuff as directed.

Hemming

On fine fabrics, you can turn under 5mm/¼in and then turn up the remaining hem allowance and slipstitch, but for heavier fabrics it would be better to neaten the raw edge with zigzag stitch and then hem, without making the extra turn.

For most of the clothes shown here it would be best to hem by hand, but the nightshirts and the shirt could just as well be topstitched with an ordinary machine straight stitch.

Neatening

Some fabrics hardly require neatening but in most cases it is better to finish off the raw edge of seam allowances by oversewing with zigzag stitch or by trimming them with pinking shears. Always neaten the free edge of facings with zigzag stitching (*see diagram*).

Finishing off a facing

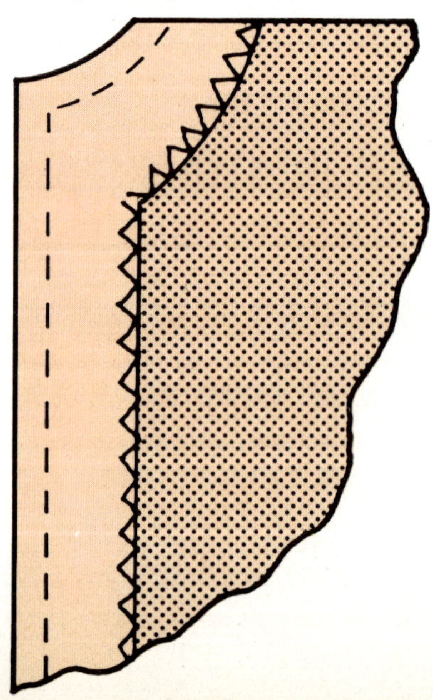

Pressing

If it is at all possible, have a well-padded ironing board and iron nearby as you sew and press each seam open (unless otherwise directed) as soon as you have sewn it.

In the case of curved seams (such as that on the nightshirt) it may be necessary to remove some of the fullness in the inner curve by taking out small notches of fabric at regular intervals along the curve (*see diagram*), while on outer curves you may have to clip the seam allowance up to the seam in order to get it to lie perfectly flat.

Clipping the seam allowance

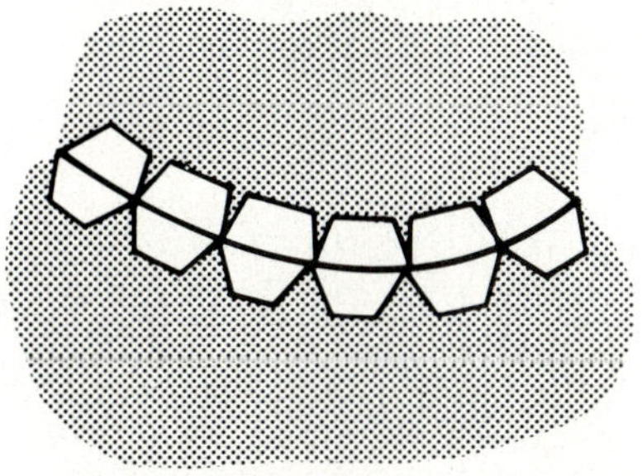

Reinforcing corners

Several of the patterns shown here have sharp corners, either at the neckline, or on collars, or at the armpit. It is a good idea to reinforce these corners by making a double line of stitching at these points. Use ordinary straight stitch and stitch in the seamline for about 2cm/¾in on either side of the corner. There is no need to finish off the ends; they are held by the finished seamline.

If the fabric is to be turned out, for example on the collar of the shirt (*page 25*), make a cut diagonally across the seam allowance at the corner so that it will lie flat.

Cutting the corners

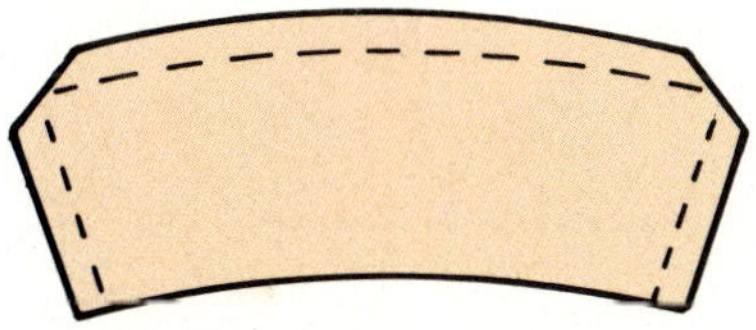

If it is an inner corner, for example the armhole of the pinafore or the jerkin, take out a notch so that there will be no excess fabric when the facing is turned round to the inside.

Appliqué

The appliqué numbers on the sportsman's nightshirt and the patchwork coat and the patches on the tailcoat (*pages 20/21, 28/29 and 30/31*) can easily be sewn on with a machine, using zigzag stitch.

You could draw the numbers directly on to the fabric if you are confident, but it would probably be easier to make templates. Draw the shapes on thin card (you can use old breakfast cereal boxes) then cut them out.

Place the templates on the fabric, if possible with the grainlines running in the same direction as on the main fabric. (In other words, do not place your templates diagonally on the fabric as this will give the patches more stretch than the fabric on to which they will be sewn, so you are likely to get more wrinkles and puckers.) Draw round each template with a well-sharpened colored pencil and cut out with sharp scissors.

Cutting out . . .

Fig 1

. . . and sewing on numbers

Fig 2

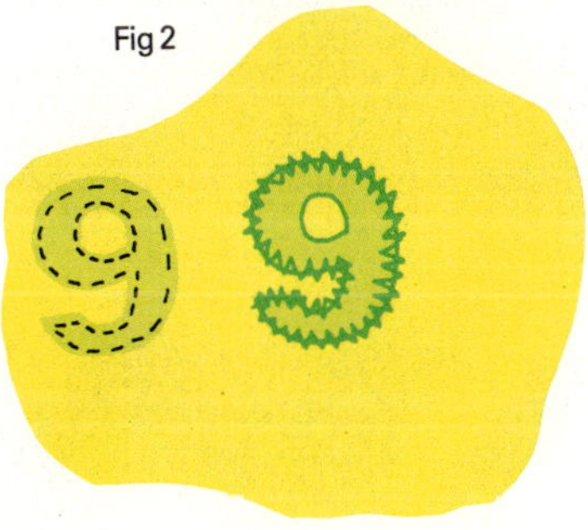

Pin the patches to the main fabric, adjusting them until you are completely satisfied with the positioning, then pin and tack them in place. It is important to tack thoroughly, otherwise puckers will tend to form during stitching. If you tack close to the edge of the patches, you will cover the tacking with your zigzag stitching so there will be no need to unpick it.

When all the patches have been tacked, sew them in position with zigzag stitch. Begin and end with a few back stitches and set the machine at a close zigzag stitch. Hold the fabric flat with your hands but do not stretch it. Do not make the stitches too close together or you will clog the machine.

When you have finished, go over the work with a sharp pair of embroidery scissors and snip off any loose ends of thread or raw edges which stick out beyond the stitching.

Slipstitching

Insert the needle upwards into the turned-over hem, 3mm/⅛in from the edge. Pull the thread through, then pass the needle down and up through the main fabric, picking up only two or three threads. Repeat procedure, keeping the stitches as even as possible.

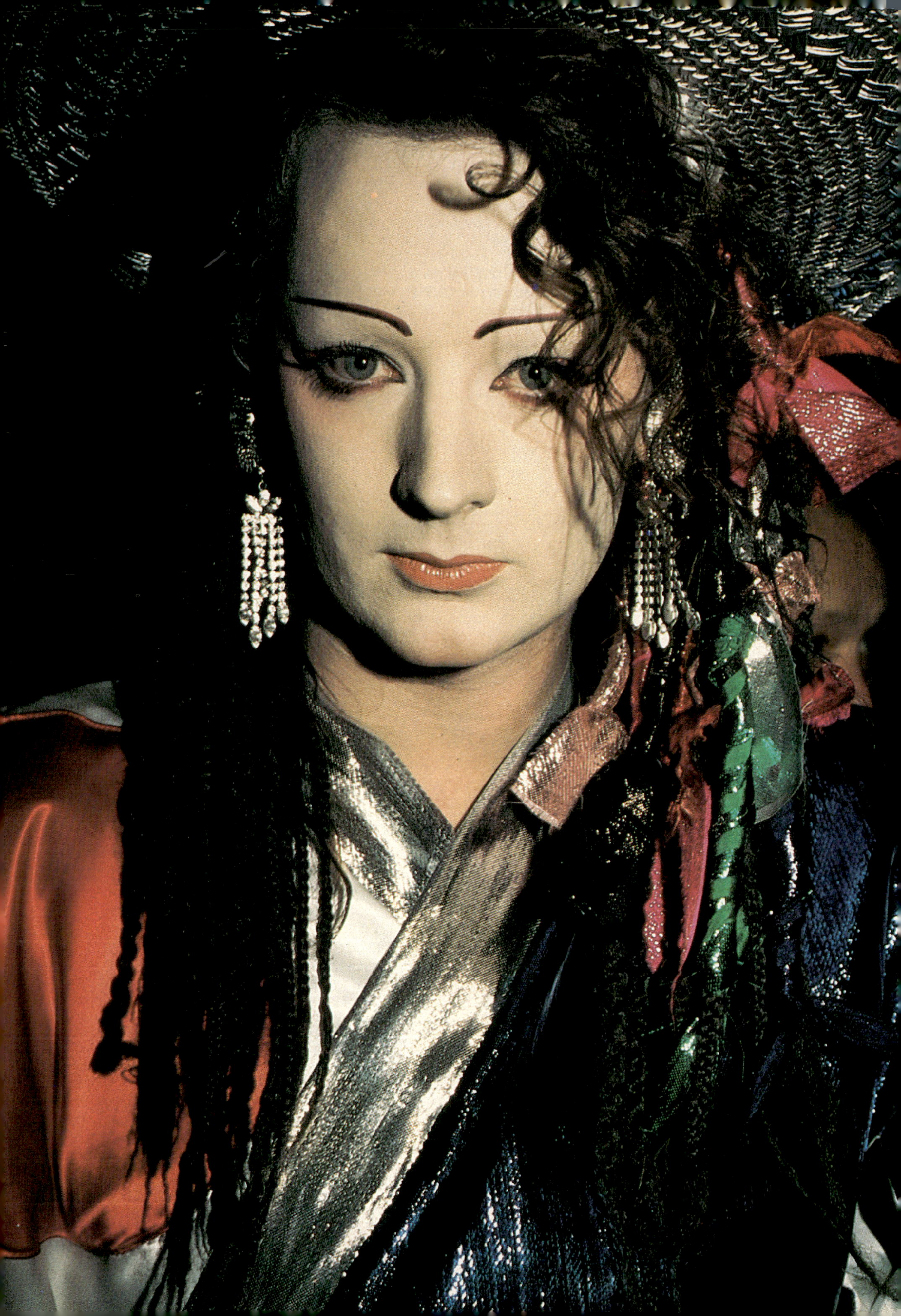

GLAM & GLITTER

The sparkle and glitter are reminiscent of the glam rock fashions worn by David Bowie as Ziggy Stardust, Roxy Music, and the New York Dolls in the 1970s. If you do not want to make the kimono featured here, it is possible to jazz up an old dressing-gown, as most men's dressing-gowns are a kimono shape: just appliqué bright strips of lurex (available from most fabric shops) on to the collar and shoulders. You can also cut small strips of lurex (or use ribbon) and tie them in your hair as George has done. ***For the hat, see page 35.***

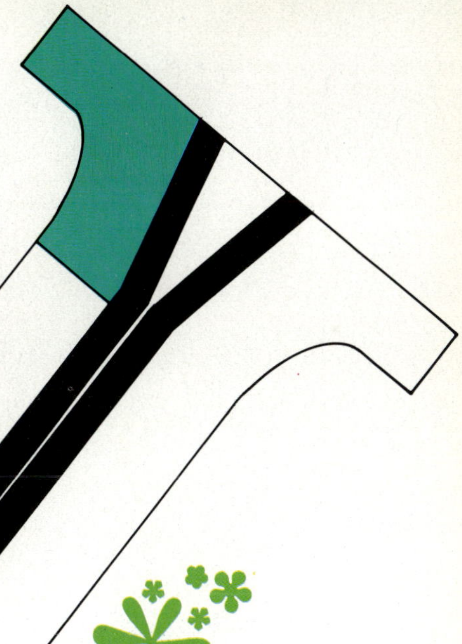

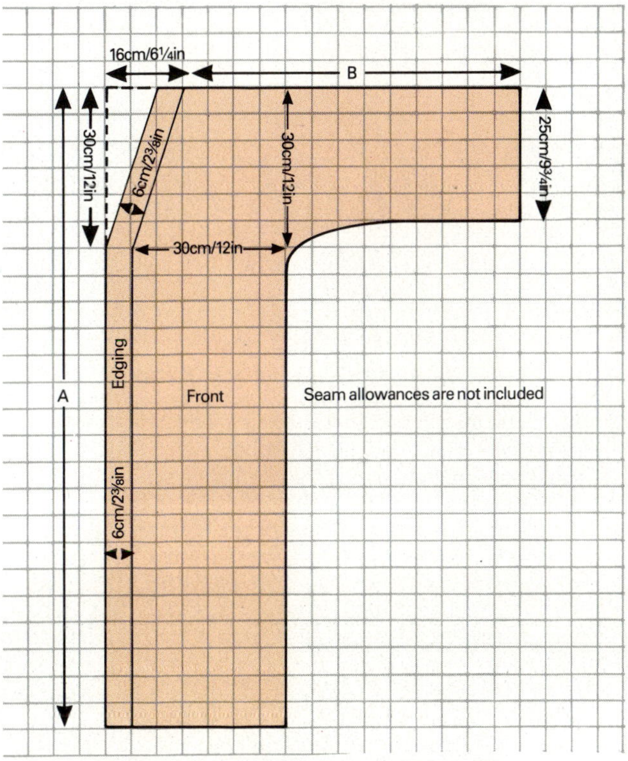

The kimono
This is one of the easiest garments in the world to sew, and even with the contrast edging and the shoulder patch this can still be made with great speed.

Materials
4m/4⅓yd (approximately, depending on your measurements) of 150cm/60in-wide fabric.
1m/1yd of 150cm/60in-wide fabric for the front edging.
Fabric for the contrast patch (use your pattern to work out how much you will need).
1 reel of thread.

The pattern
Start by measuring from your shoulder down to mid-calf, to give measurement A. Then measure from a point 6cm/2⅜in in from the edge of your shoulder and down to your wrist, to give B.

Draw a horizontal line across the top of your paper measuring B plus 16cm/6¼in, and a vertical line (A) down from the left-hand corner. Draw a line parallel to line A and 6cm/2⅜in away from it, up to a level 30cm/12in below line B, then draw a horizontal line 30cm/12in long. This line marks the top of the side seam (start of the underarm curve).

Complete the front and edging pattern pieces, following the measurements given on the diagram. Add 1.5cm/⅝in seam allowances and 4cm/1½in at the hem. To make the shoulder patch simply draw a line across the front pattern piece, just below the start of the V-neck, then trace off the top and bottom pattern pieces, remembering to add 1.5cm/⅝in seam allowances at the join.

The back pattern should measure twice B plus 36cm/14¼in at the shoulder. Use the front pattern to draw the wrist edge and side/underarm lines, then just draw a line across at the bottom (if you follow this method, seam allowances will then be included).

Making the kimono
Cut out the top and bottom front pieces and join them, then cut out the matching front piece. Cut four front edgings (two pairs) and the back.

Setting a pair of edging strips to one side, join the remaining edgings to the fronts. Press the seams towards the edgings, clipping into the stitching line at the angle if necessary.

Join the fronts to the back at the shoulder, leaving 1.5cm/⅝in free at the neck edge. Neaten the back neck edge and turn in the seam allowance, catch-stitching to hold it in place.

Join the side/underarm seams.

With right sides together, attach the remaining edging (facing) strips to the front, stitching across at the hemline, then bring them round to the back. Turn the seam allowance under and slipstitch the facings in position. Hem round the bottom of the kimono.

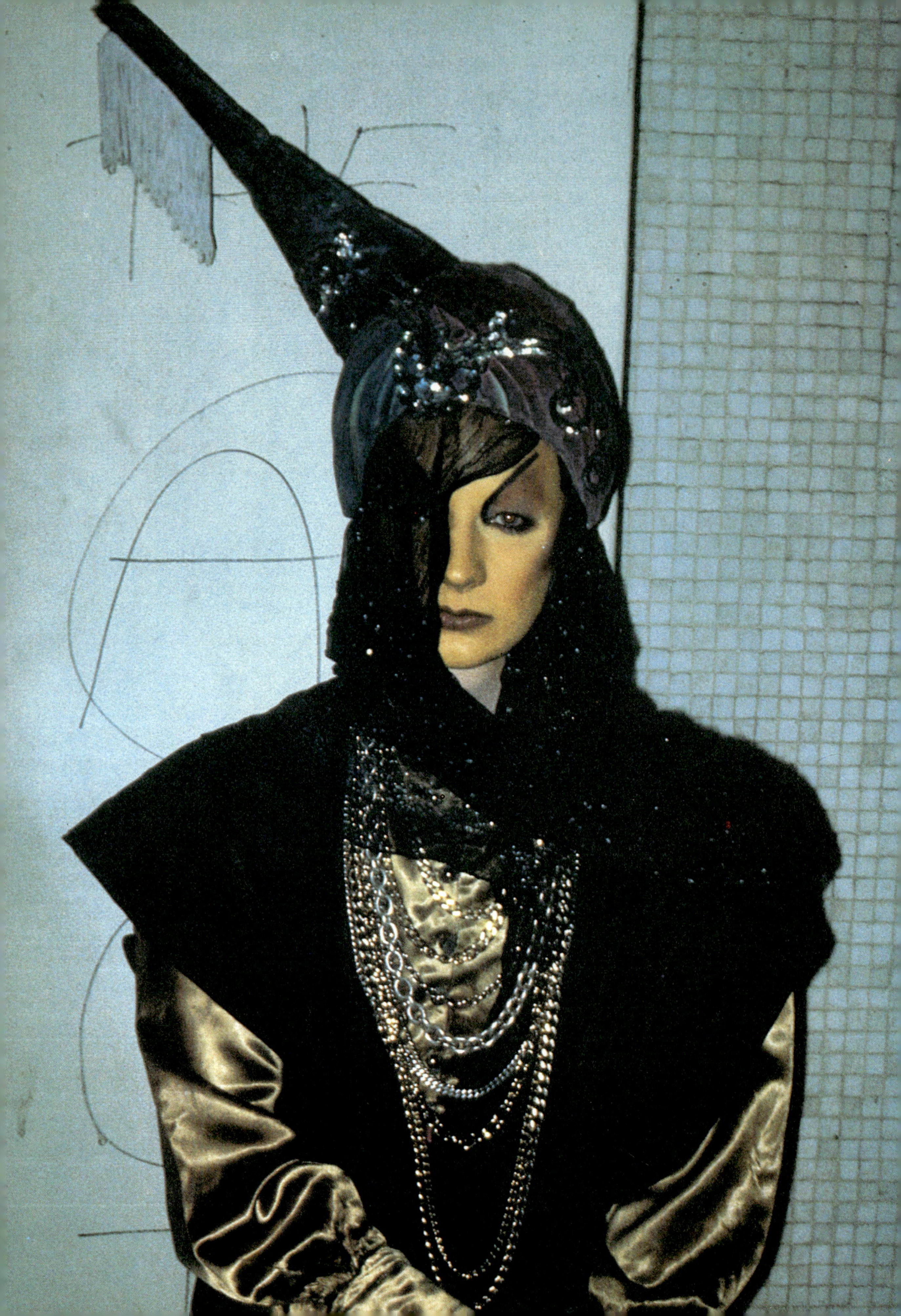

DESERT PRINCE

Boy George's dress sense is the result of combining many separate styles into his own, highly individual cross-culture dress. Here he combines the look of a desert prince with the futuristic shapes of a Darth Vader outfit.

The hat looks expensive, but is in fact very easy to make (*see page 35*). The shirt worn under the jerkin can be obtained by raiding your mother's wardrobe. George gives the finishing touch to his outfit with a set of chain necklaces. This, again, is easy to make: use different lengths and thicknesses of chain (these are available in brass or a silver color from hardware shops) and hold them together at the back of the neck with pins.

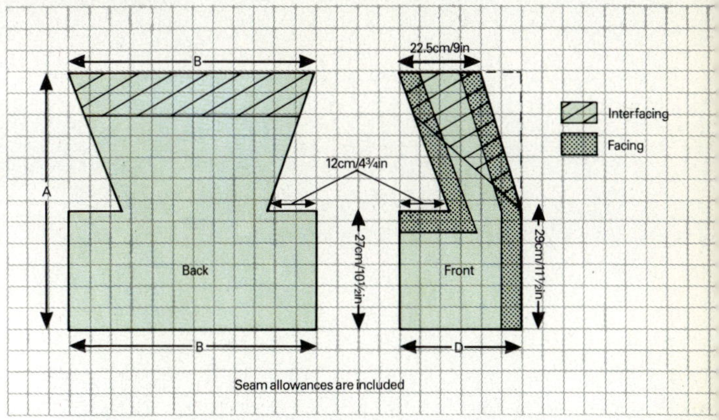

Jerkin

This jerkin is one of the simplest patterns in the book – basically it is just two oblongs sewn together, with a V-shaped cut at the front and triangles taken out at the sides to make the armhole shaping. You can use a quick and easy iron-on interfacing to give the stiff, angular shape at the shoulders and if you are in a hurry, you can forget the facing and just hem round all the edges.

Materials

Approximately 1.5m/1⅔yd of 90cm/36in-wide or 70cm/27½in of 150cm/60in-wide black cotton fabric or light-weight wool (the amount will vary considerably according to your measurements and the width of the fabric).
Interfacing.
Black thread.

Note You can use iron-on interfacing or the sew-in kind (*page 10*), depending on how much time you have to spare and whether you want to wash the garment frequently. The iron-on type will tend to pucker a little with frequent washing. Do not choose too stiff an interfacing or you will tend to see a line across the chest at the point where it finishes.

The pattern

Start by measuring from your shoulder down to about 2cm/¾in below the point of your hip bone and add 6.5cm/2½in to make measurement A.

For measurement B, measure from shoulder to shoulder and add 20cm/8in (the jerkin juts out 10cm/4in from each shoulder plus 3cm/1in for seam allowances). Measurement C is half of B less 7.5cm/3in (for example if B is 60cm/23½in, C will be 30-7.5=22.5cm/12-3=9in), while D is half B less 5mm/¼in.

Make your front and back pattern using these and the measurements given on the diagram.

To make the interfacing pattern, lay the front pattern piece shoulder to shoulder with the back pattern, matching the seamlines so that the seam allowances overlap. Trace off one side (back and front together), then flip the front pattern over to the other shoulder and repeat for the other side, so that the interfacing pattern is all one piece (the points will overlap slightly at the front, but only a small amount of seam allowance will be lost, which does not matter).

Make a front facing pattern (6cm/2⅜in wide) and armhole facing pattern to the shaded areas.

Making the jerkin

Cut two fronts and a back, four (two pairs) of armhole facings, a pair of front (neck edge) facings and a strip measuring 27cm/10½in by 6cm/2⅜in for the back neck facing. Cut these from the main fabric. Also cut the interfacing from the interfacing fabric.

Join the fronts to the back at the shoulder and the front (neck) facings to the back facing strip. Also join the armhole facings at the shoulder. Press the seams open.

Neaten the outer edge (the edge farthest away from the neck edge) of the neck facing and do the same for the armhole facing.

If you are using an iron-on interfacing, iron it in position. If you are using the sew-in kind, stitch it in position round the neck edge and armholes (1.5cm/⅝in seam allowance). Join the side seams on the main garment.

With right sides together, stitch the neck facing to the main garment, turn it in and press. Reinforce (*page 11*) the corners of the armholes on the main garment, then with right sides together, stitch the armhole facings to the main body. Turn the facings in, clipping as necessary, and press.

Finish by hemming (5cm/2in hem allowance) round the bottom edge.

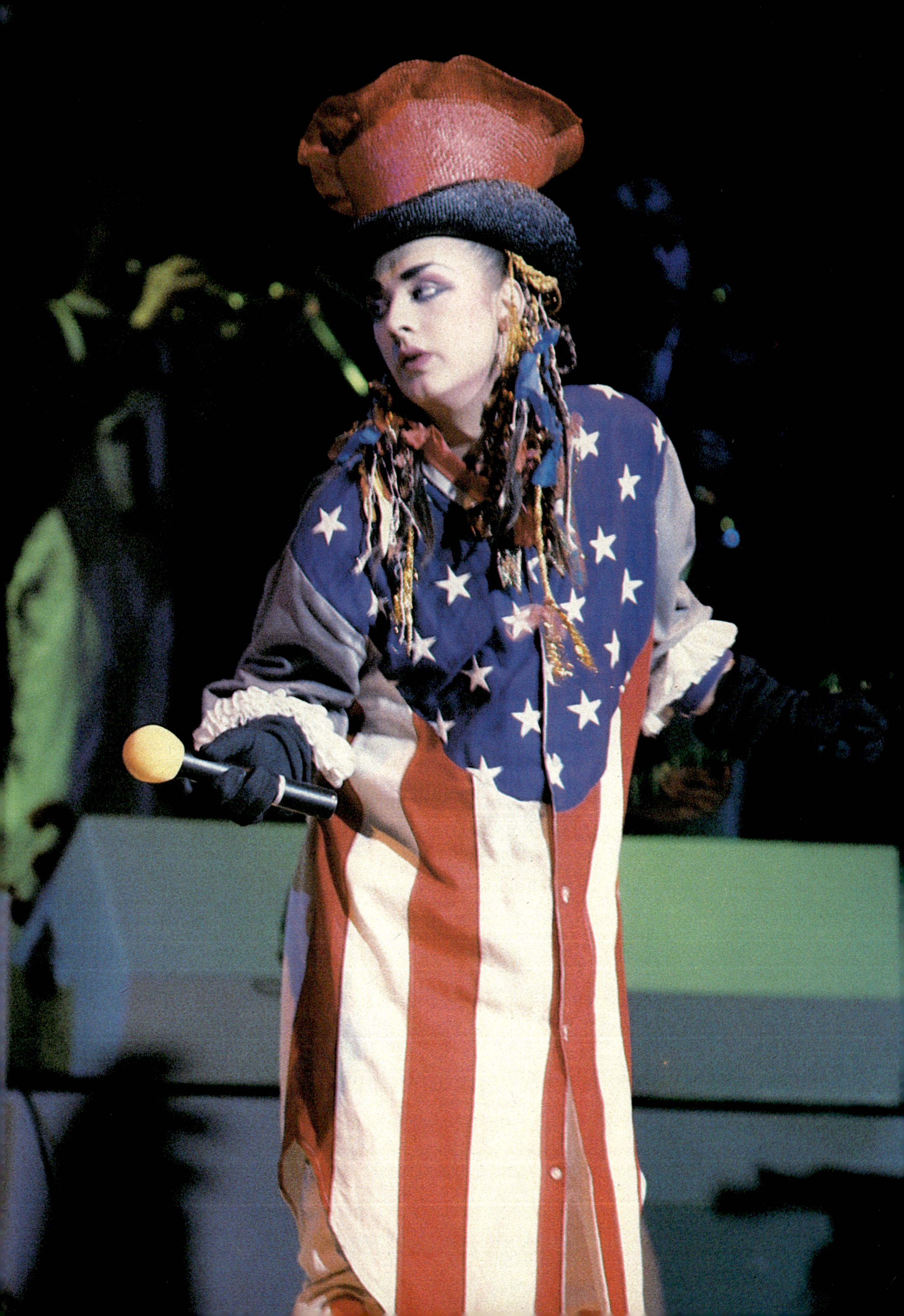

YANKEE DOODLE DANDY

George sings the praises of the USA in his Mad Hatter outfit. This is a little more difficult to put together than many of his other outfits, but nevertheless it can be done.

His hat is based on that worn by the Mad Hatter in *Alice in Wonderland* by Lewis Carroll, and is made of painted straw. You can quite easily make your own version however (*see page 34*).

The fabric of the stars and stripes nightshirt might be difficult to find and expensive to buy, but you can achieve a similar effect if you are willing to experiment.

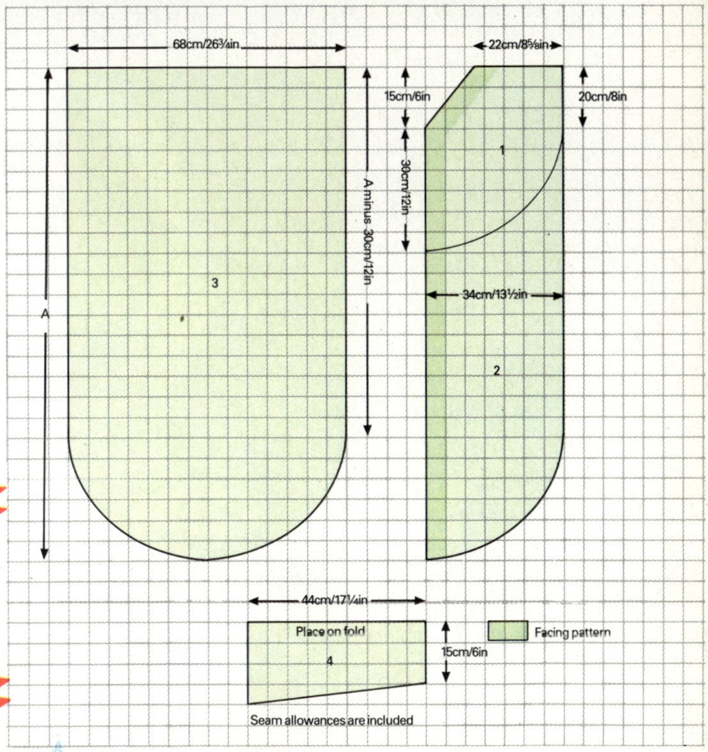

Nightshirt

The nightshirt is easy to make but the fabric is hard to find. Maybe you know someone who has an old flag; otherwise you may have to settle for some polka-dot fabric to replace the stars, and perhaps a fabric with narrower stripes for the bottom section and the back.

Materials

1m/1yd of 90cm/36in-wide medium-weight star or polka-dot fabric.
2.5 or 3m/2⅔ or 3⅓yd (depending on your measurements) of 90cm/36in-wide medium-weight striped fabric.
1m/1yd of 90cm/36in-wide medium-weight plain fabric.
1.2m/1¼yd of white lace trim.
7 x 2cm/¾in-diameter white buttons.
2 reels of white thread.

The pattern

There are four main pattern pieces: a top front section, a bottom front section, a back and a sleeve.

Start by drawing the side front (pieces 1 and 2) as one piece (you cut along the yoke line to make the two sections at a later stage). First measure the length from your shoulder to mid-calf (A); note that the side seam is less 30cm/12in.

Using measurement A and the other measurements given, draw a complete side front section. Use a bent wire coat hanger to draw the bottom curve.

Next draw the back, using the front piece as a guide, flipping it over along the centre front line to draw the second side and taking the line straight across at the top. Add 1.5cm/⅝in all the way round.

Again using a coat hanger, draw the curve at the front yoke and cut along the curved line. Re-draw both pieces, adding 1.5cm/⅝in seam allowances except on the yoke curve (add 1cm/⅜in).

Use the front pattern pieces to make 7cm/2¾in-wide facing patterns (see the shaded area on the diagram), and cut a strip measuring 38cm/15in by 7cm/2¾in for the back neck facing.

Finally, use the given measurements to make the sleeve pattern, adding 1.5cm/⅝in allowances at the wrist edge, armhole and underarm seams.

Making the nightshirt

Cut two sleeves, placing the top arm line on the fold, from plain fabric. From the striped fabric, cut one back and a pair of bottom fronts (pattern piece 2). Cut a pair of top fronts (pattern piece 1) from polka-dot fabric. Cut one back facing and two of each of the front facings from the appropriate fabrics.

Join each top section to its corresponding bottom section along the curved seam (1cm/⅜in allowance). Also join the top and bottom front facings.

Now join the fronts to the back at the shoulders, and do the same with the facings.

Cut the 1.2m/1¼yd of lace in half, run a gathering thread through the top of each lace strip and add a gathered frill to each sleeve edge. To do this, turn under the seam allowance at the sleeve edge, pull up the gathering thread until the lace strip is the same length as the sleeve edge, pin and tack it under the folded edge (make sure the gathers are even) and top-stitch right through all the layers.

Attach the sleeves to the main body along the armhole seam.

Stitch the side and underarm seams. Neaten the inner, non-seam edge of the facing and, with right sides together, stitch the facing in position all round the front edge, then turn it in to the wrong side and press.

At evenly spaced intervals, make seven buttonholes and attach buttons to correspond. Make the hem, turning under 5mm/¼in and then 1cm/⅜in.

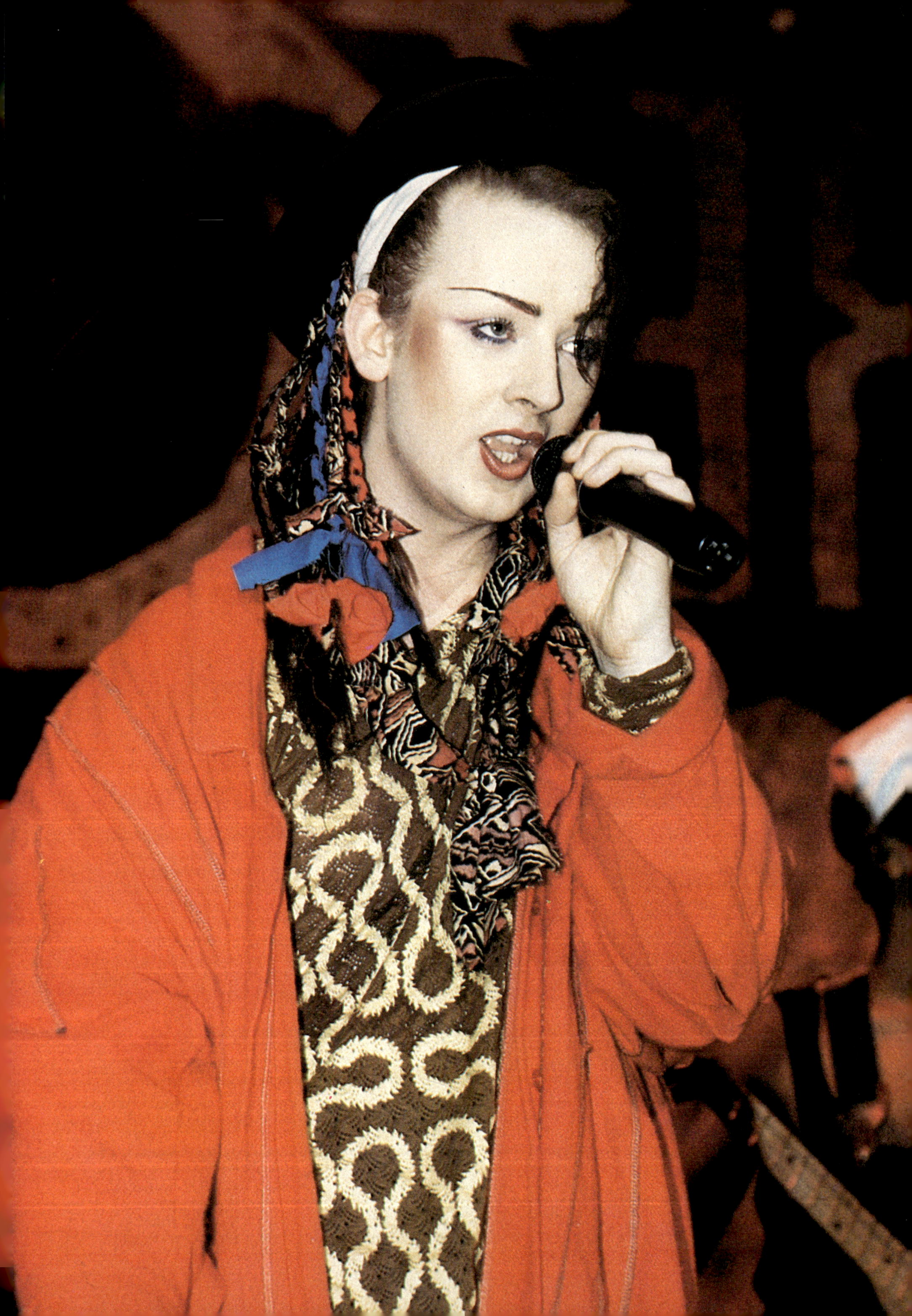

RED REBEL

George in his African ethnic outfit. His coat and shirt both come from top London designers and are consequently very expensive; however, as with most of his outfits, they can be made comparatively cheaply.

The look is, as usual, very much exaggerated and vividly colored. The coat is large and stitched in a contrast thread, giving it an unfinished look. The shirt is shaped like a sack and can be made using the same pattern as that given for the 'tailcoat' (*page 31*), but without the tail.

Alternatively, African or Indian caftans can be bought, but they tend to be expensive. The scarf is a small piece of ethnic print fabric simply knotted round the neck. The hat can be an old bowler hat or a trilby with the top dent pushed out.

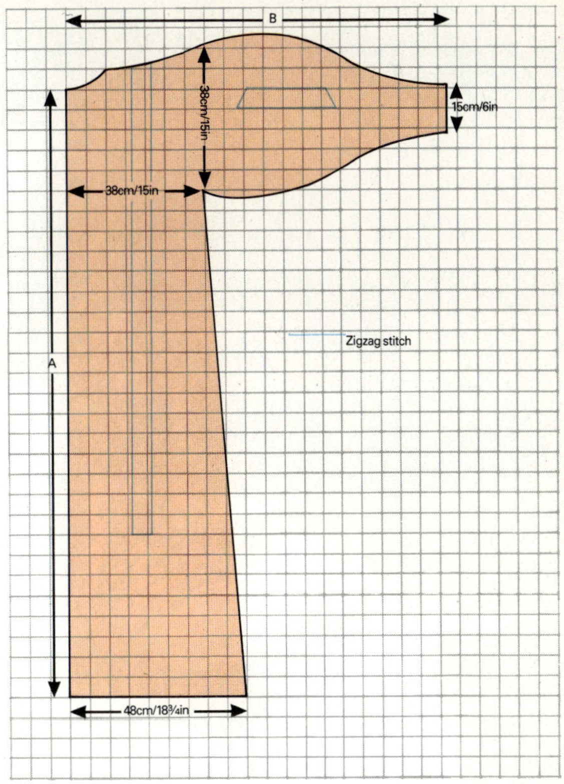

Ethnic coat
The coat is very dramatic and eye-catching but quite easy to make, being formed from one pattern piece repeated four times, with a straight collar added.

Materials
4⅓ or 5m/4⅔ or 5⅓yd of 120cm/45in-wide medium- or heavy-weight bright red cotton or linen.
2 reels of white thread.

The pattern
Take the following measurements: from the hollow of your neck to your ankle and add 1.5cm/⅝in (A), and from the hollow of your neck to your wrist. Add 14.5cm/5¾in to this to give B. Draw up the pattern to these and the other given measurements (this also includes 1.5cm/⅝in seam allowances).

Make a shallow shaping at the neck and use a bent wire coat hanger as a guide when making the arm shaping.

The collar pattern is made in the same way as that of the nightshirt (*page 21*) and should be cut 15cm/6in wide (this also includes 1.5cm/⅝in seam allowances).

Making the coat
Cut four pieces (two pairs) from the fabric, dovetailing them to save fabric (*see page 9*). Cut one collar. Using white cotton and zigzag stitch, make lines of decorative stitching as indicated on the pattern.

Join the four pieces together along the shoulder, side and centre back seams. Zigzag stitch round the front edges, the wrist edges and the bottom edge of the coat. Fold the collar in half lengthways, right sides together, and stitch across the ends. Turn it right way out and with right sides together, attach it to the coat down one long edge. Fold the other long edge under and then catch-stitch it in place.

Finally, cut two strips of fabric 40cm/15¾in long and 3cm/1in wide to tie round the wrists, giving the coat its billowed-sleeve effect. You can either neaten the strips with zigzag stitch or leave raw edges.

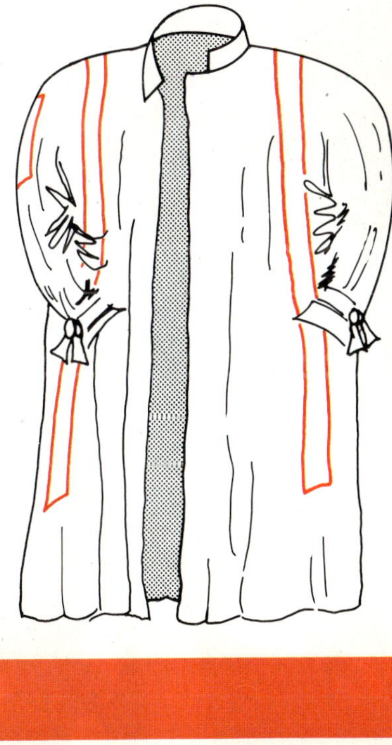

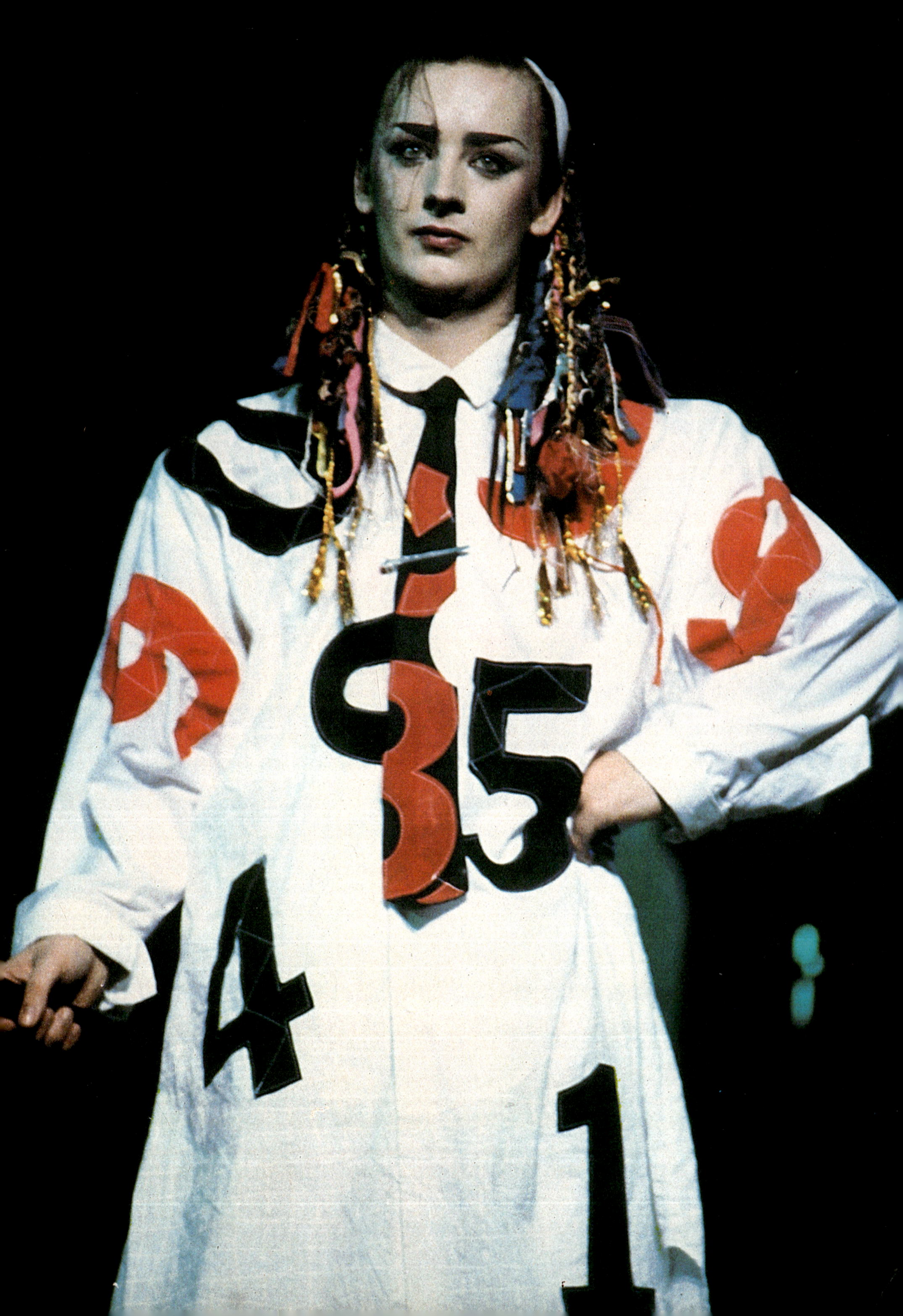

NIGHT NUMBERS

A simple nightshirt and long-johns are transformed into a sporty outfit by the imaginative use of numbers.

George's penchant for exaggeration is to be seen in the vast size of the nightshirt and the numbers. By wearing the enormous shirt over narrow leggings and adding eye-catching shocking-pink socks, George gives the outfit three distinct layers – layering being one of the most fashionable ways of dressing in the 1980s. You can use crisp white cotton or an old bedsheet to make the nightshirt, or alternatively your father or grandfather might have one hidden away somewhere. The socks and shoes can be bought from sports shops.

If you cannot find the socks, buy white pure cotton or pure wool socks and dye them.

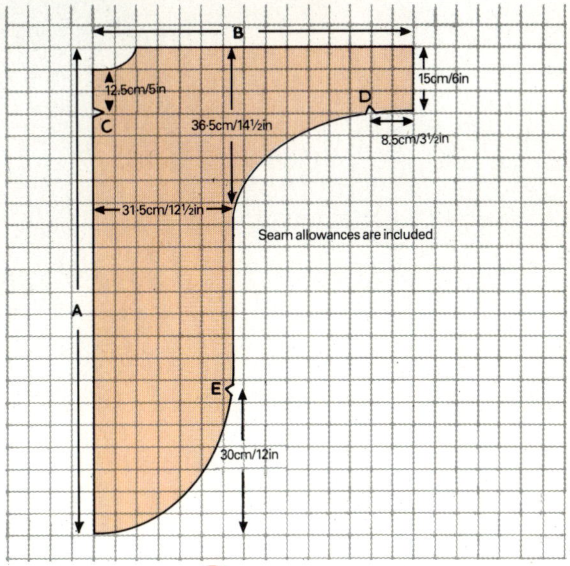

Sportsman's nightshirt

This is made from three main pieces (a back and two fronts) and three small ones (a simple straight collar and cuffs), with red numbers appliquéd on.

Materials

3 or 4m/3⅓ or 4⅓yd (depending on your size) of 150cm/60in-wide medium-weight white cotton fabric.
1.5m/1⅔yd of 90cm/36in-wide red cotton fabric (it must be colorfast).
1 reel of white thread.
1 reel of red thread.
2 x 1.5cm/⅝in diameter red buttons.

The pattern

Take the following measurements: from the hollow of your neck to just below the knee and add 3cm/1in to give the centre front length of the shirt (A), and from the centre back of the neck along your outstretched arm to the wrist, again adding 3cm/1in to make length B.

Now draw one front pattern piece, using your own and the given measurements.

Shape the neck in a shallow curve and make a note of the measurement of the curve on the stitching line (1.5cm/⅝in in from the cut edge). Mark notches at C (12.5cm/5in down from the neck edge), D (8.5cm/3½in in from the wrist edge) and E (30cm/12in above the bottom level).

To obtain the curve under the arms and at the tail, bend a wire coat hanger to the required shape and draw along it.

For the back, just turn in the seam allowance down the centre front of the front pattern, draw round one side, flip the pattern over (keeping the centre front in the same position) and draw round the other side.

For the collar, multiply the noted neck measurement by four, add 3cm/1in (seam allowances) and make a pattern to this length and 9cm/3¾in wide. The cuff pattern should be drawn 14cm/5½in long and 6cm/2⅜in wide, with a curved edge at one end.

Making the nightshirt

Cut a pair of fronts, one back, one collar and two cuffs, placing the short straight edge of the cuff piece on a fold so that each cuff measures 29cm/11½in. Cut numbers from the red fabric.

Using red thread and zigzag stitch, appliqué on all numbers which do not overlap two pattern pieces, then join the fronts to the back at the shoulder/top arm seams and complete the appliqué.

Turn in the centre front seam allowances at the neck edge. Fold the collar lengthways, right sides together, and stitch across the ends.

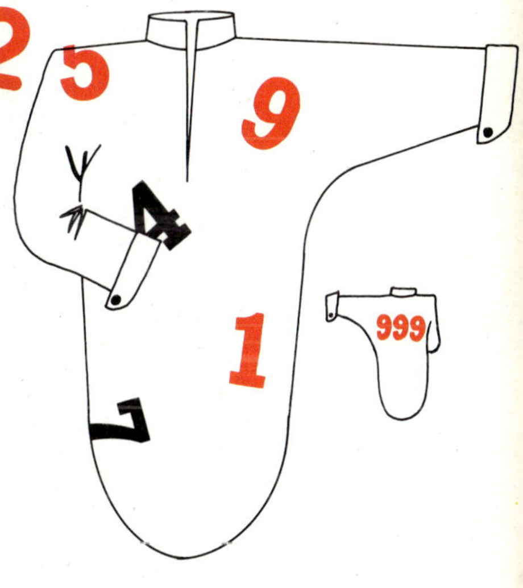

Turn it right side out. With the right sides together, attach the collar to the neck edge down one long side. Turn under the seam allowance down the other long side and catch-stitch it in place. Join the side/underarm seams from D to E. Turn in the (underarm) seam allowances from D to the wrist edge. Stitch the cuffs to the sleeves, leaving an overlap of 2cm/¾in at either end.

Join the centre front from C to the bottom. Hem round the bottom edge of the shirt, then make a narrow hem (turning in 5mm/¼in, then 5mm/¼in again) round the cuffs.

Catch-stitch the seam allowances in place along the front opening and at the wrist.

At each cuff, make a buttonhole and sew a button to correspond.

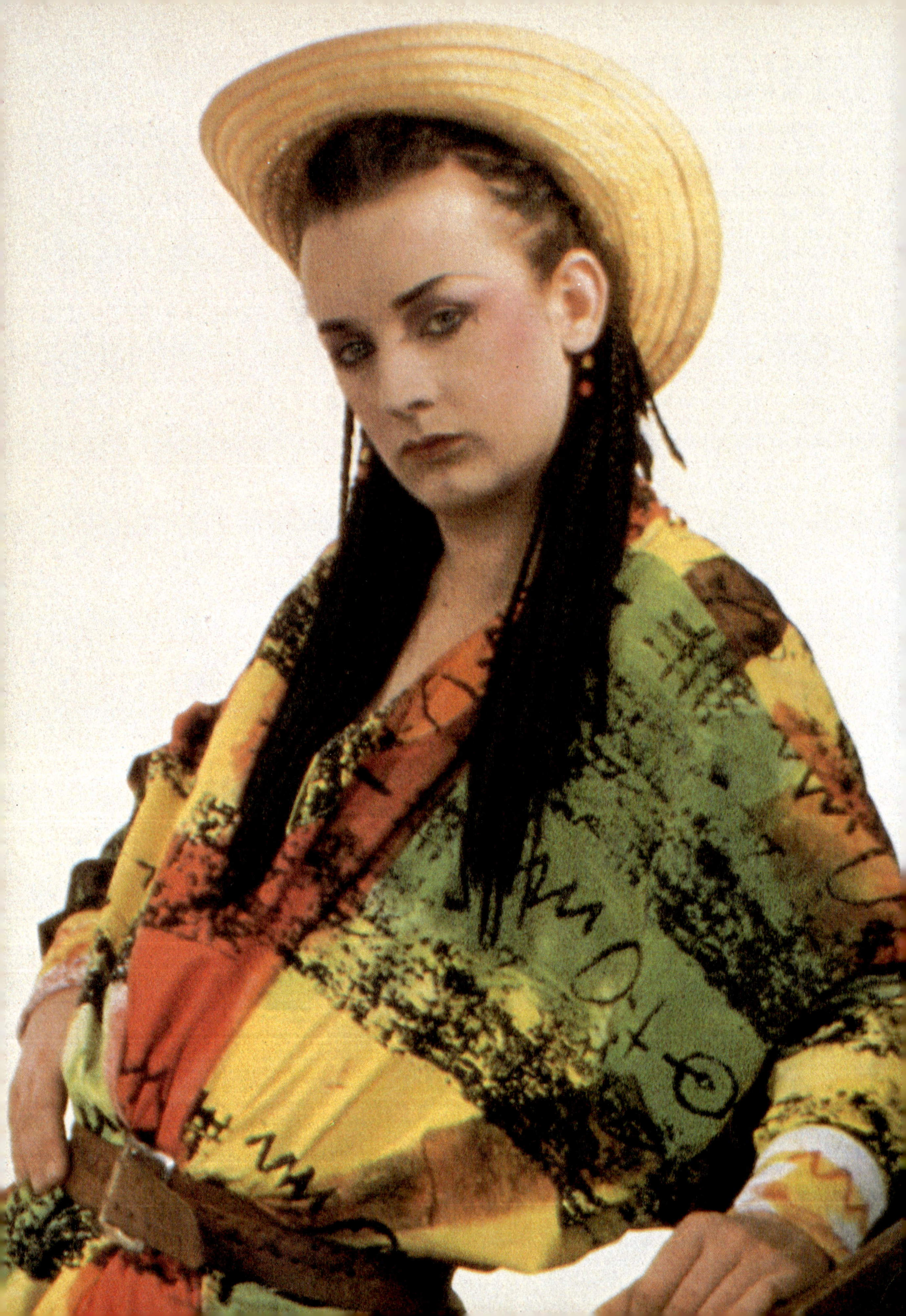

GORGEOUS GRAFFITI

When Culture Club first became popular, this was the outfit that Boy George wore most frequently. The prints and clothes are both the work of a young London designer, Sue Clowes. The writing and symbols are copies of graffiti left by tramps and hobos on the walls and pavements of London at the turn of the century.

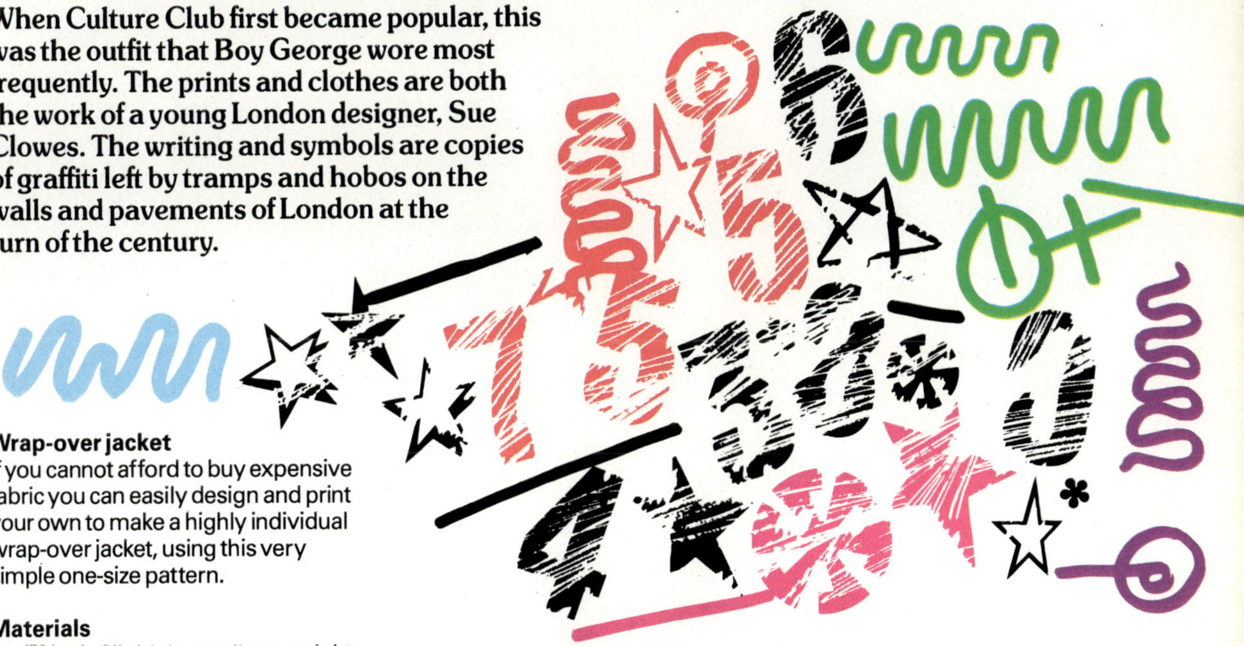

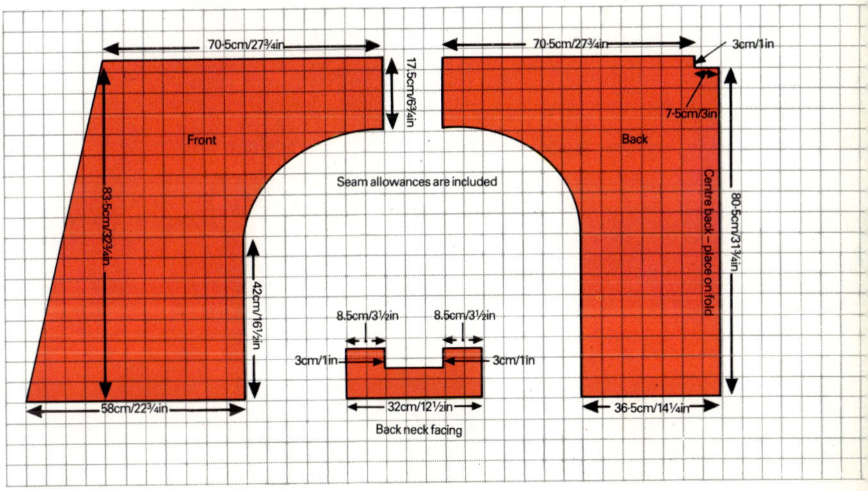

Wrap-over jacket

If you cannot afford to buy expensive fabric you can easily design and print your own to make a highly individual wrap-over jacket, using this very simple one-size pattern.

Materials

3m/3⅓yd of light- to medium-weight brightly-colored plain cotton fabric.
Fabric paints.
Sponge.
Potato.
Masking tape.
1 reel of thread.

Dyeing the fabric

Try to find a pure cotton fabric because natural fibres, such as cotton or linen, dye more easily than synthetic ones. You will find fabric paints, which can be painted directly on to fabrics, in craft shops.

Stretch the fabric over a padded surface such as a table covered with an old blanket or a (washable) work-top. (You may find that you have to print a section at a time.) Secure it with masking tape.

The rough-tyre print that runs right across George's jacket can be fairly effectively recreated by dipping a sponge lightly into a saucer of dye (do not let it get too wet), and dabbing it on the fabric.

Individual shapes and signs can be painted on (use a variety of brushes, including old decorating brushes) or you can use the potato-printing method to good effect.

For potato printing, cut a potato in half, sketch your design on the flat, cut surface of one half with a point and whittle away the flesh around it so that the design stands out. Dip into a saucer of dye and apply.

When you have finished the printing, place paper over the fabric and press with a hot iron.

Making the jacket

Using the given measurements, which include seam allowances of 1.5cm/⅝in, and 2cm/¾in at the hem and sleeve edges, make the front and back pattern pieces and the back facing pattern.

Use a bent wire coat hanger to make the curve then copy the side seam from one pattern piece to make the other.

Cut out two fronts and one back piece, placing the centre back on a fold. Cut out the back facing and neaten it down the two (11.5cm/4½in) side edges and the long edge.

Attach the fronts to the back at the shoulder/top arm seam, leaving 1.5cm/⅝in free at the neck edge. Join the side/underarm seams.

With right sides together, attach the back neck facing to the back, matching the un-neatened edge to the back neck edge. Turn the facing to the inside and catch-stitch it in place along the shoulder seam.

Check the length and trim the sleeves or the bottom hem if necessary, then hem round the sleeve edges and bottom hem, turning up 5mm/¼in and then 1.5cm/⅝in, and the front edges (5mm/¼in and 1cm/⅜in), mitring the points at the front.

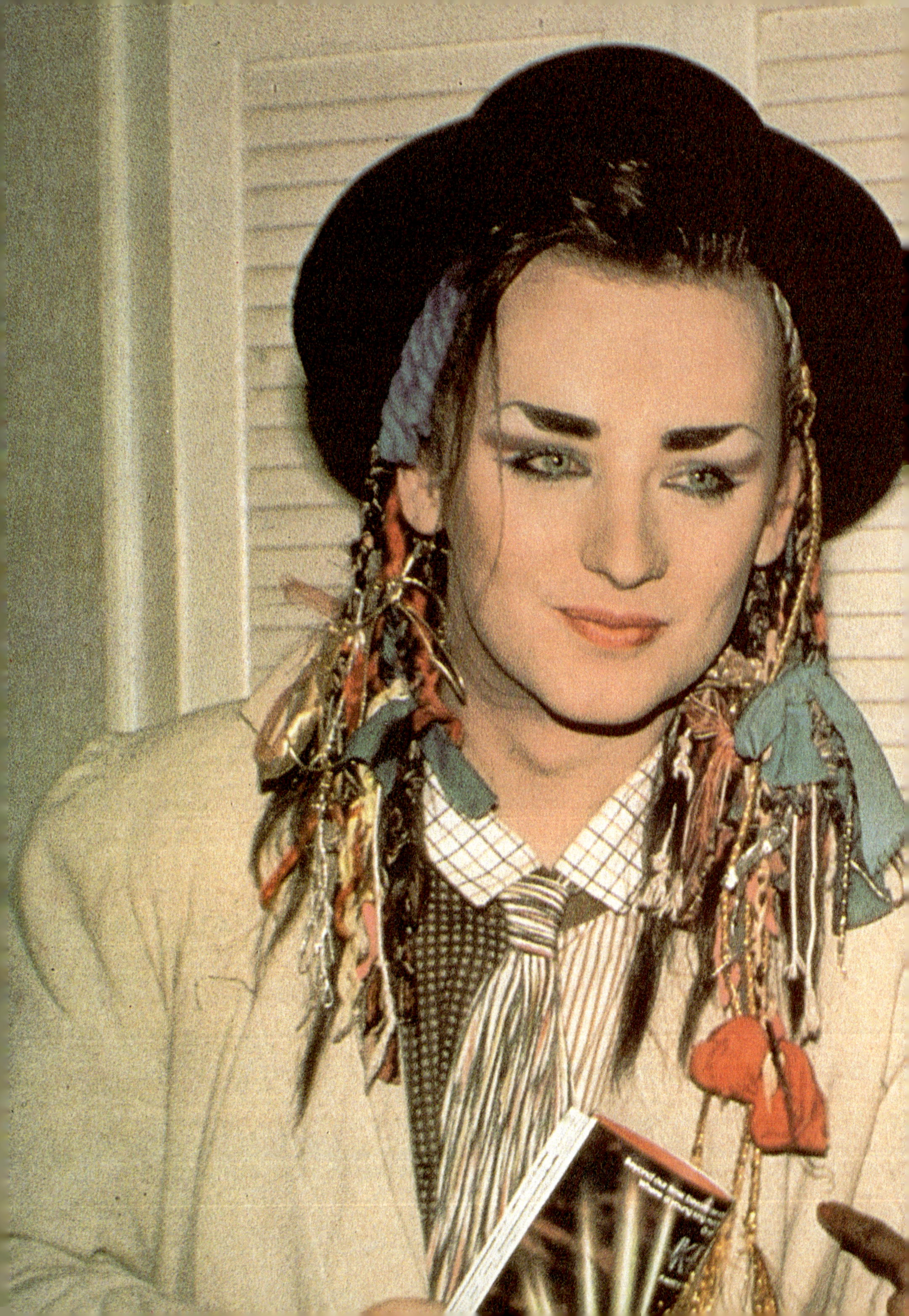

PATCHWORK GANGSTER

Boy George seems to be dressing in a traditional way for once (disregarding his hair of course!), but his smart jacket-shirt-and-tie look has a difference – the sleeves, fronts, collar, cuffs and back of the shirt are a patchwork of three separate fabrics.

The tie can be any brightly-colored tie, or even a colorful strip of fabric (cut it 1m/1yd long by 4cm/1½in wide). The jacket is a 1940s double-breasted gangster-style one, of a kind which are available in the more fashionable mens-wear shops but which are, unfortunately, expensive.

If you make the usual round of attics, jumble sales and so on, however, you should be able to find one somewhere. George is again wearing his favorite hat, the pushed-out trilby (*see page 35*).

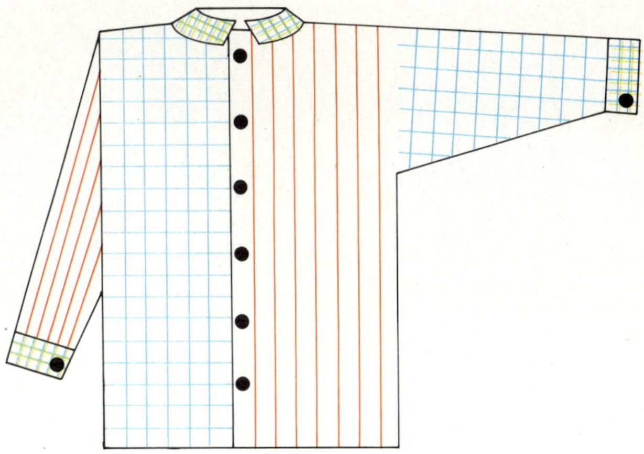

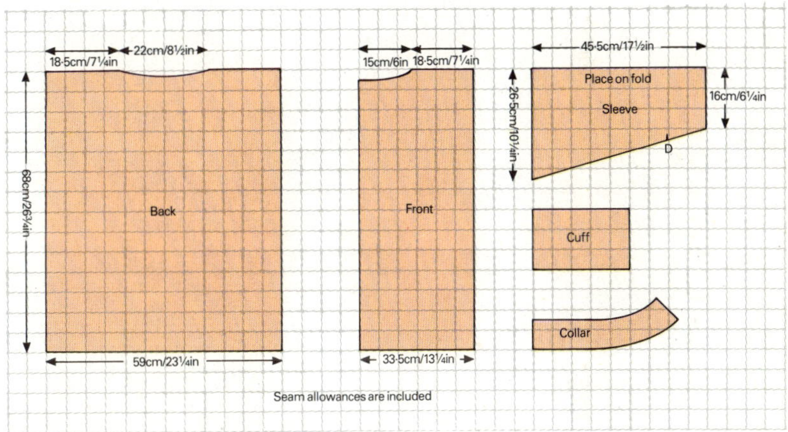

Multi-colored shirt

The shirt looks complicated because of the patchwork effect, but in fact it is very easy to make – just a matter of cutting the main pieces from three different fabrics.

Materials

3 × 1m/1yd lengths of 90cm/36in-wide lightweight cotton fabric in coordinating colors – A, B and C.
1 reel of thread.
8 buttons.

Making the shirt

The pattern given above is a single size one for people with a shoulder span of up to 56cm/22in. If you require a larger shirt, leave the sleeves, cuff and collar patterns and the neckline of the shirt as they are but add 5cm/2in to the shoulder, length and width measurements of the front and back.

Scale up the pattern (1 square = 5cm/2in) and cut as follows: one sleeve and one shirt front from fabric A and the same from fabric B, then two collars, two cuffs and the shirt back from fabric C. Note that seam allowances of 1.5cm/⅝in are included throughout.

Start by neatening the raw edge down each centre front (use zigzag stitch or oversew by hand) then join the fronts to the back along the shoulder seams. Then, with right sides together, fold back 2cm/¾in down the centre front on each front piece and stitch across at the neck edge. Clip in to the end of the stitching line as shown on the diagram, turn the fold right side out and press.

With right sides together, sew the two collar pieces together, leaving the shorter (inner) curved side open. Turn the collar out and press.

Holding the collar open, and with right sides together, pin and tack one side (this will be the undercollar) in position on the neck edge, then stitch. Turn under the seam allowance on the remaining free edge, clipping as necessary, and slipstitch it in position on the neck edge.

Join the sleeves to the main body of the shirt and stitch the side/underarm seams up to D, leaving them open from D to the wrist edge. On the remaining 9cm/3¾in, turn the seam allowance under to the wrong side (first 5mm/¼in then 1cm/⅜in) and then proceed to hem.

Next make two 3cm/1in deep tucks in the sleeve edge, with the folded edge of each tuck lying 2cm/¾in from a (hemmed) side seam. Tack the tucks to hold them in correct position.

With right sides together, fold each cuff in half lengthways and stitch across the short ends, then turn the cuffs right side out. With right sides together, pin each cuff to a sleeve edge down one long side. Stitch and then fit the other long side over the sleeve edge, turning in the seam allowance and slipstitching it in to required position.

Hem round the bottom edge of the shirt and make eight evenly-spaced buttonholes.

Finally, sew on buttons to match.

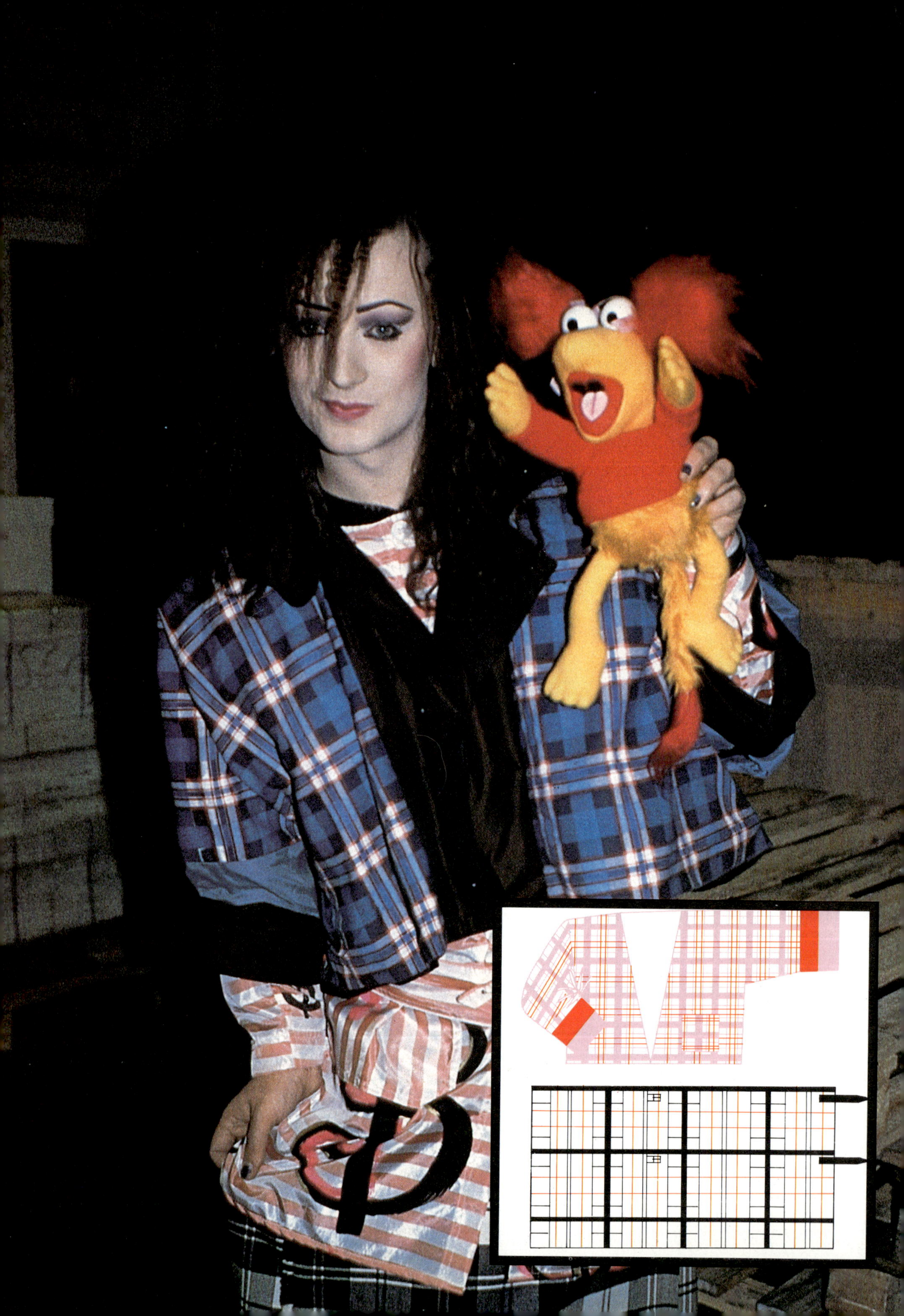

HIGHLAND REEL

In George's Scottish outfit, a simple kilt and tartan bolero jacket is worn with a cleaner's overall covered with dollar signs. The multi-layered look is very evident: George even wears two pairs of traditional Scottish socks, plaid socks being worn under thick woollen walking socks.

Both of these can be purchased from traditional menswear shops, while the kilt can be bought from specialist shops or you can make one yourself. For the striped overall, or something similar, try your mother's cleaning cupboard.

You can draw dollar signs on an ordinary apron, using an indelible marker pen. The shirt and tartan bolero worn over the apron make, including the socks, six visible layers.

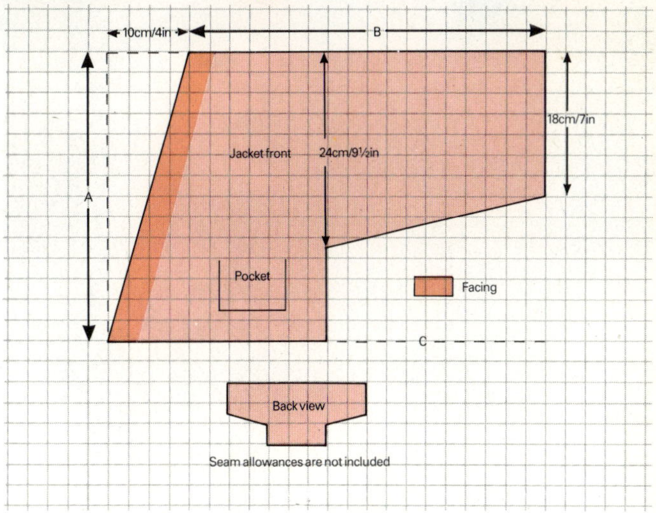

Jacket and kilt

The short bolero jacket has two bands of contrasting fabric at the sleeves, and patch pockets. The kilt is made from a single strip of fabric wrapped round and could be worn over trousers or thermal underwear.

Materials

For the jacket:
1.5m/1⅔yd of medium-weight tartan or check fabric (120cm/45in or 150cm/60in wide, depending on your measurements).
20cm/8in strip from each of two contrast fabrics.
1 reel of thread.
For the kilt:
50cm/20in of 120cm/45in-wide medium-weight tartan or check fabric.
1 reel of thread.
2 buckles and leather straps to match.
1 hook and eye.
1 kilt pin.

The jacket pattern

Take the following measurements: from the top of your shoulder to your waist (A) – the length of the jacket – and, with arm outstretched, from the neck edge to a point about midway between wrist and elbow (B).

To make the jacket front pattern, draw a line across the top of your paper and another at right angles to it down the left hand side. Mark measurement A on the vertical line, and draw another horizontal line (C) at this point. On the top line, mark a point 10cm/4in in from the left and another point measurement B farther along, to make the shoulder/top arm seam. Draw from the start of line C up to the 10cm/4in point to make the front edge of the jacket.

Measure from your neck edge to a point 5cm/2in beyond the edge of your shoulder and mark this measurement on the pattern. Draw a faint vertical line from here down to line C. The side seam starts 24cm/9½in down this line. The sleeve edge should measure 18cm/7in, giving you the angle of the underarm seam.

Positioning the pocket

Mark the position of the pocket on the front pattern. The finished pocket is an oblong 15cm/6in across and 13cm/5in deep. The bottom line of the pocket should be 6cm/2½in above the hem and one side should be 13cm/5¼in away from the side seam.

The back jacket is the same as two fronts without the neck shaping and without the pocket placement mark. The shoulder line of the back should measure twice B plus 20cm/8in.

Add a 4cm/1½in hem allowance at the bottom of both pieces and a 1.5cm/⅝in seam allowance the rest of the way round.

Make a front facing pattern to the shaded area shown on the pattern (the facing should be 8cm/3¼in wide at the shoulder, including the seam allowance). Cut a strip of fabric measuring 33cm/13in by 8cm/3¼in for the back neck facing.

Making the jacket

Cut two fronts and a back, two front facings, a strip measuring 33cm/13in by 8cm/3¼in for the back neck facing, and two oblongs of fabric measuring 18cm/7in by 18.5cm/7¼in (depth of pocket plus turn-ins) for pockets.

Start by neatening the top edge of each pocket, then turn under the top 4cm/1½in and hem. Turn in a 1.5cm/⅝in allowance round the other edges of each pocket and tack (you will have to trim the corners so that they fold down neatly). Place the pockets in position on the jacket fronts and topstitch down the sides and along the bottom, 1cm/⅜in in from the folded edge.

Join the shoulder seams on the main pieces and the facings, then neaten the inner, non-seam edge of the facing.

Cut two 10cm/4in-wide contrast bands, one in each colour for each sleeve, and sew them in position.

Join the side/underarm seams.

With right sides together, join the facing to the main body all round the neck and front edges. Turn the facing to the inside and catch-stitch it in position. Hem round the bottom and sleeve edges.

The kilt

No pattern is needed for this. Simply make 2cm/¾in-deep hems along both cut edges (waist and hem). Wrap the kilt round to see where to fasten the buckles, one at the waist and one about 20cm/8in down. Attach the hook and eye to hold the inside corner in place.

Girls may want to make four tucks at the back, to shape the waist. Make sure that they are even and top-stitch them for about 7.5cm/3in, down from the waist edge.

For a finishing touch, secure the overlap with a kilt pin.

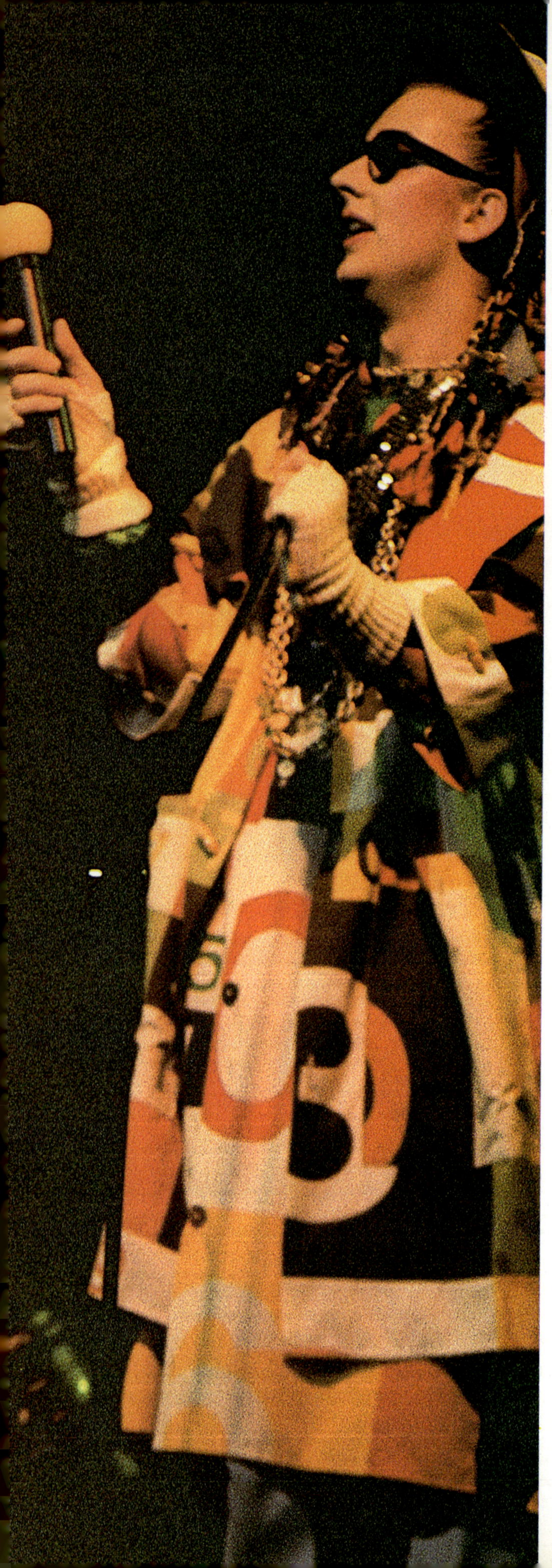

NUMBER GAME

This is an outfit to make anyone stand out from the crowd, highlighting many parts of the body.

A huge black straw hat draws attention to George's head (if you cannot find a black one, you could spray-dye an ordinary straw hat). His fingerless gloves attract the eye to his hands and arms – you can buy these or, preferably, cut the fingers off an old pair of ordinary gloves. But dominating everything else is the coat. You most certainly cannot buy one of these in any ordinary shop but if you are willing to try, you will find that it is surprisingly easy to make your own.

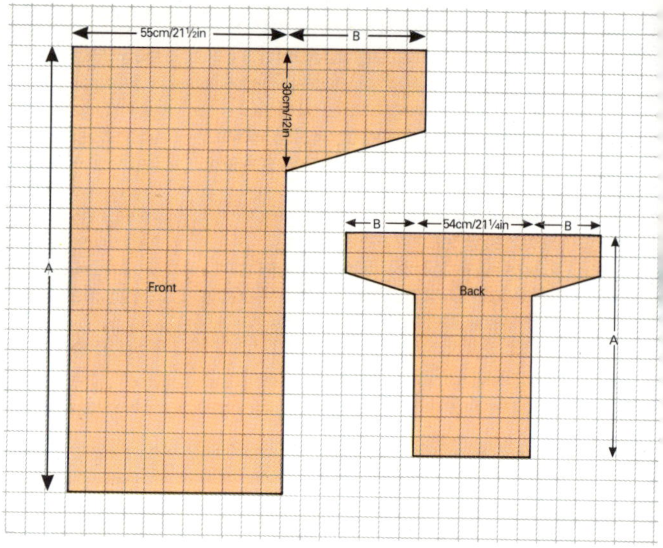

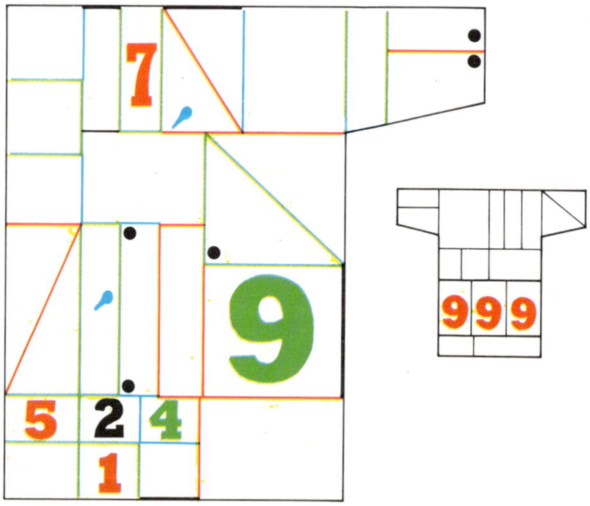

Patchwork coat
George's maximum-impact coat takes a little more time to make than some of the other clothes shown here but is basically very simple – just three pattern pieces – and designing the patchwork is fun, while the sewing can be done very quickly with a machine.

Patchwork materials
The amount of fabric needed will vary greatly according to your size and to the patchwork pattern which you design. What is required is a selection of plain fabrics (you could of course have some with geometric patterns if you want) in a large range of colors. It is best to choose all medium-weight cotton or all wool because different fabrics tend to shrink differently, resulting in a crumpled effect. It would also be best to make your pattern and sketch out your patchwork design before buying the fabric, so that you can decide how much is needed of each color.

In addition to the patchwork fabrics you will, if you decide to bind the edges of the coat rather than just hemming it, need enough of one fabric to make the binding (*see Binding*).

The coat can be decorated with buttons, toggles and beads sewn on at random.

The design
Start by making scale drawings on graph paper of the back, left and front outlines, using the measurements in the diagram. Measurement A is the length from your shoulder to mid-calf. The coat has an off-the-shoulder sleeve, so for the sleeve (measurement B) measure from 10cm/4in off your shoulder to a point midway between your wrist and elbow. The length of the top line of the pattern for the back should be twice B plus 54cm/21¼in.

The next step is to settle down with the graph outlines, a pencil, a ruler and a set of colored pencils and listen to your favorite Boy George numbers as you design your own patchwork pattern, using the basic style of the coat shown in the picture. This is a big, bold coat, so don't make any of the patches too small and fiddly. The design shown in the photograph is composed of squares, triangles and rectangles of varying sizes, with numbers appliquéd on at random. You could either choose numbers or your own personal symbols and hieroglyphs.

Use colored pencils to shade in the outlines of the patches and go on experimenting and playing around with different combinations of colors until you are really satisfied with the design. (It is a good idea to check first that the colors which you want to use are available, otherwise you might have to dye neutral-colored fabric.)

Make your design one which can easily be sewn by machine, checking that patches always meet side on and that no patches jut into each other.

Making the patchwork
When you are happy with your design, spend a while looking at it and deciding how you are going to join it up. The method with this kind of patchwork, where there are patches of varying sizes, is to join triangles into squares, small squares into rows and the rows into blocks, progressively making the patchwork blocks larger and larger until the work is completed.

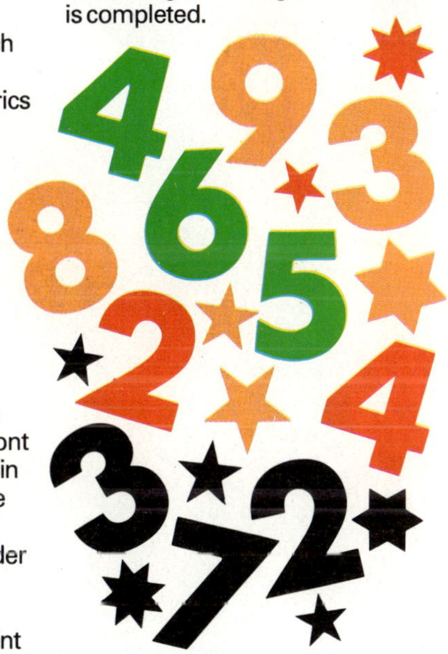

Sizing the shapes
The next stage is to work out how large your patches should be, using the graph paper to scale them up and adding 5mm/¼in seam allowances all round each patch. Using a ruler, pencil and set square, draw the patches on the appropriate fabrics then cut them out.

It helps to pile the patches in each separate block together so that you do not have a lot of tedious sorting out to do when you sew.

If you are putting numbers or other symbols on some of the patches, the next stage is to work the appliqué, as it will be much easier to sew them on at this stage.

When all the patches are prepared and in the relevant piles, stitch them together, using a neutral-colored thread. This sounds time-consuming but it need not be: the loose ends of thread will be secured by the succeeding patches so there is no fiddly finishing off to be done.

If you find it difficult to keep to a 5mm/¼in seam, a useful tip is to stick a strip of masking tape 5mm/¼in away from the needle hole on the base plate of your machine and use this as a guide (*see page 10*).

When you have sewn several patches into pairs, iron the seams to one side, then do another batch of stitching and so on. Remember to use your design to show you the quickest and best order of work.

Adding strips
Start by pressing your completed patchwork pieces and then check that they are the right size. If not, don't worry, just cut them down to the right size or add extra patchwork strips.

If you are not going to bind the edges, join the fronts to the back at the shoulders then fold back 20cm/8in along each centre front (right sides together) and stitch across at the neck edge and the hem, on the stitching line. Turn the fold to the back to make a self facing and catch-stitch it in place down the centre front. Join the side/underarm seams then finish by hemming round all the remaining edges (1.5cm/⅝in allowance).

If you are going to bind the edges, join the shoulder seam then fold in a 20cm/8in allowance down each centre front (wrong sides together), making a self facing. Stitch across in the seamline at the neck edge and at the hem, then catch-stitch down the centre front to hold each facing in place. Bind the sleeve edges (*see Binding*) then sew the side/underarm seams and bind both the neck and hem edges.

Binding
If you are binding the edges, cut 10cm/4in-wide strips of fabric, joining lengths when necessary to make them long enough to go round the neck, sleeve and hem edges.

Prepare the binding strips by pressing them in half lengthways. Next, attach binding strips to the sleeve edges (right sides together) and press the seam towards the binding. Join together the side/underarm seams.

Attach binding strips round the hem and neck edges, then bring all bindings to the back of the garment and, turning under the seam allowance, slipstitch in position.

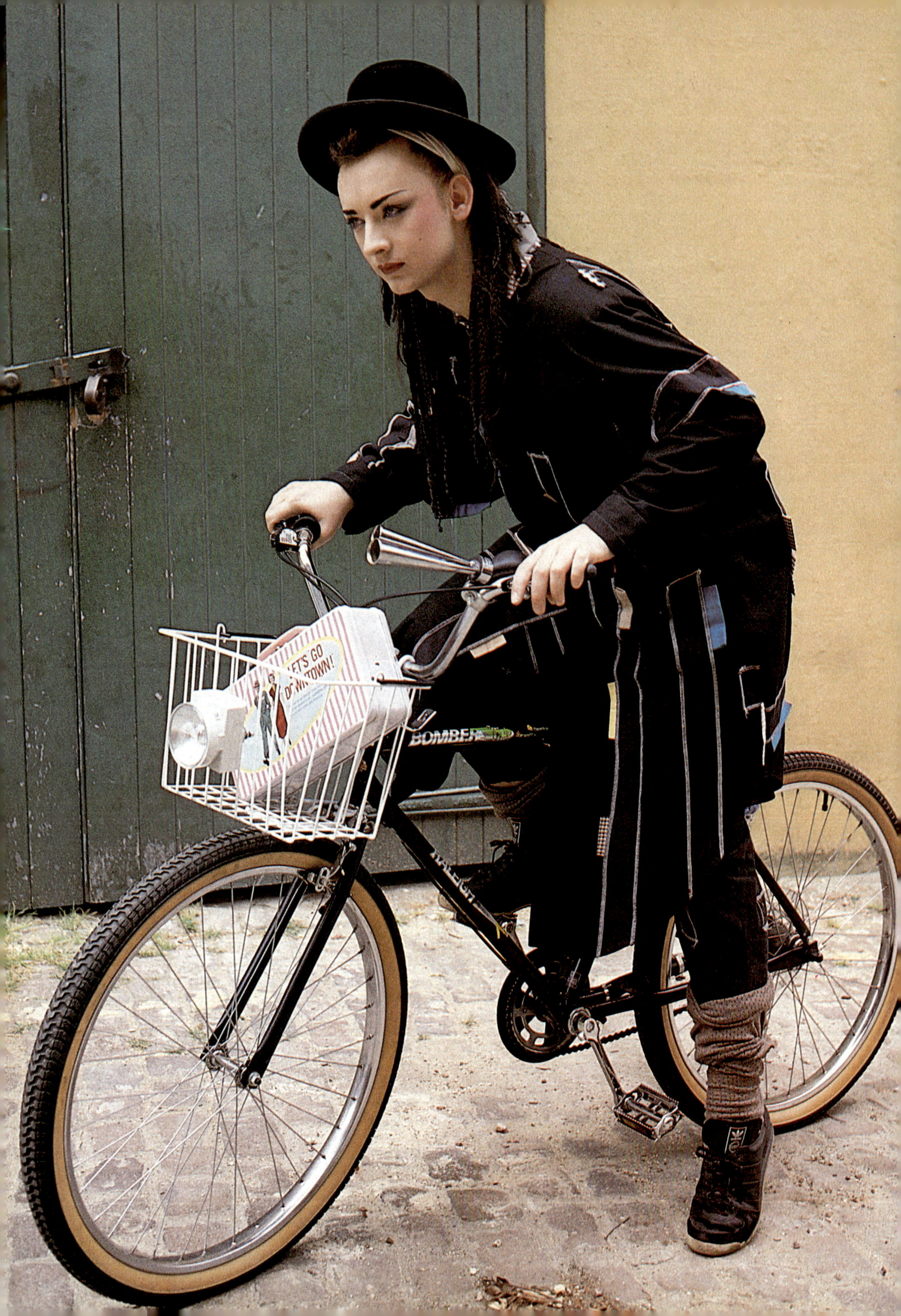
LET'S GO DOWNTOWN!
BOMBER

THERMAL STARS

George's dress sense combines traditional gents' hats, socks and even underwear with loose-fitting long coats and sportswear.

Here, George is shown riding to the recording studio in an outfit which demonstrates his cross-culture dressing superbly. His hat is simply an ordinary trilby with the top pushed out, worn with a headband. The black trousers are just thermal underwear bottoms, dyed black. Track suit bottoms would do just as well and can be bought from any sports shop, along with George's training shoes. The socks are ordinary men's socks.

The highlight of the outfit is the coat, worn with the tail falling to the front and decorated with patches and white zigzag stitching. White stitching on a black coat goes against all the rules of tailoring, but on George it looks fashionable, while the contrast patches give the coat a Dickensian, Fagin-like touch.

Tailcoat

The coat is made from just two simple pattern pieces – a back and a front – rather like a caftan. The back and front are identical except that the front is shaped down into a point and slit up to the waist to make the 'tails'.

Lines of white zigzag stitch, tabs or patches of brightly colored material and fabric bows or tassels are added.

Materials

Depending on your size, 3m/3⅓yd or 4m/4⅓yd of 150cm/60in-wide heavy cotton or linen or medium-weight wool fabric.
Scraps of bright fabric for patches and bows.
2 reels of matching thread.
2 reels of white thread.
10cm/4in of a bright, contrasting fabric for the headband.

The pattern

Start by measuring from the hollow of your neck down to the mid-calf (measurement A), to give you the length of the coat down to the point.

Then stretch out your arm and measure from the hollow of your neck down to your wrist (B). Measure your waist (C) – the finished coat will be twice as wide as your waist. Finally, measure from the top of your shoulder to your mid-chest to give the sleeve width (D).

Using these measurements and the diagram you can now make a pattern for the front of the coat. Include 1.5cm/⅝in seam allowances for the side/underarm and shoulder seams – all other edges are finished with zigzag stitch. The back is the same as the front but without the point, making it 20cm/8in shorter. You can shape the neck edge as you like, but check your head measurement to make sure that you leave an adequate, but not too large, gap.

Making the coat

Cut out the back and the front then sew on strips of brightly colored fabric at random. Use the white thread for this and zigzag stitch. You can either appliqué the patches, sewing round all sides (*see page 11*), or fold each patch in half lengthways and stitch down one side only, leaving the folded edge and the two short edges free, to make a tab.

Make lines of plain white zigzag stitch, as indicated in the diagram, then cut strips of brightly-colored fabric, form them into bows or tassels and stitch them on by hand.

Cut a slit up the front of the coat, to about waist height, and zigzag up the two edges, using matching thread. Join the back and front together along the shoulder and the side/underarm seams, then finish the neck, wrist and hem edges with zigzag stitch, once again using matching thread.

The headband

Take the 10cm/4in strip of fabric and fray the edges to give a scarf effect.

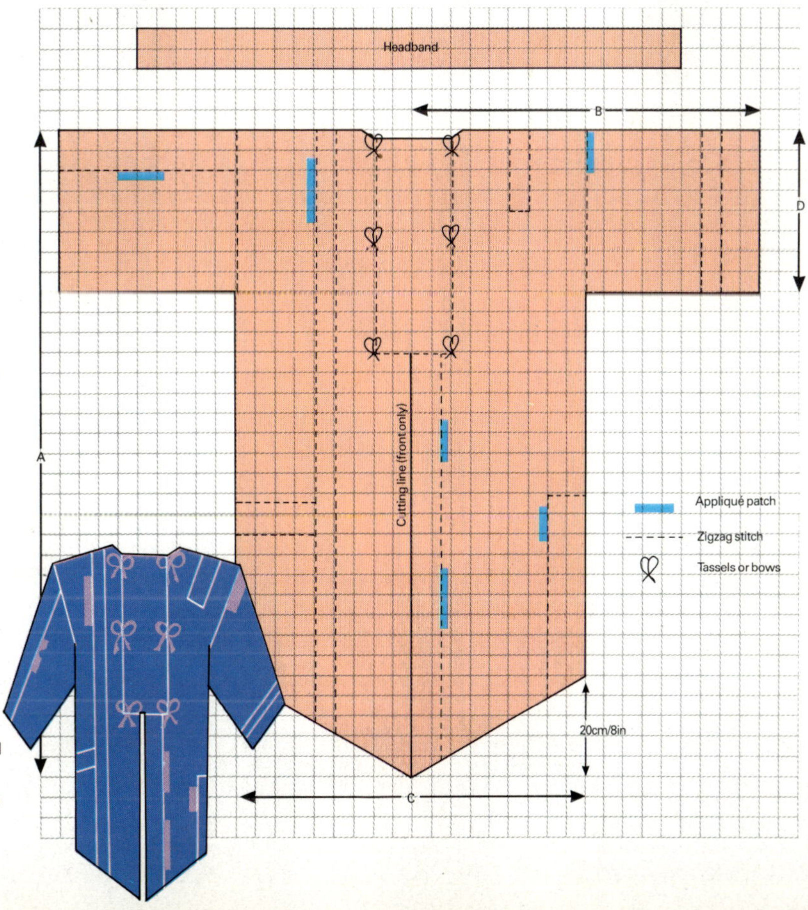

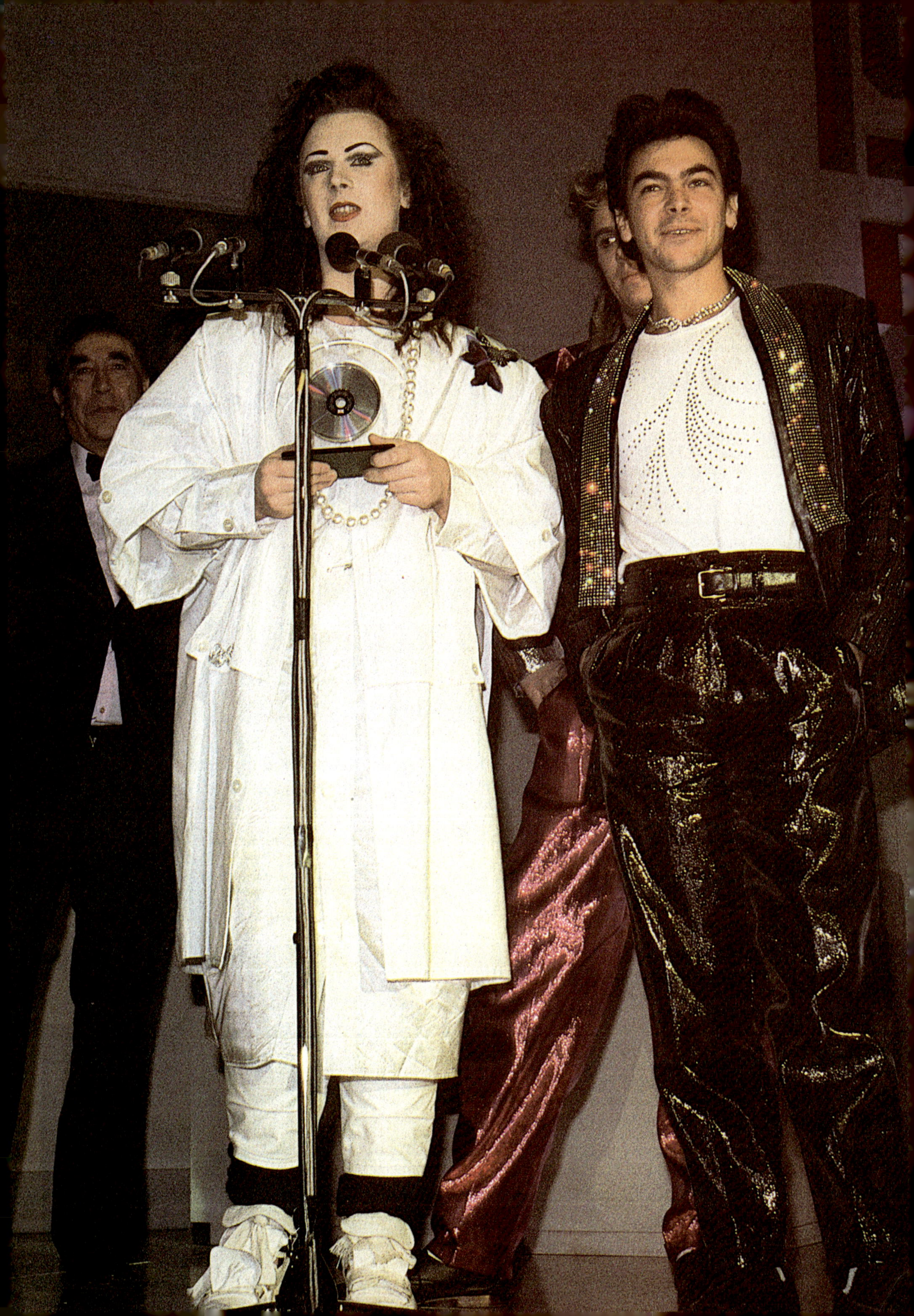

KNIGHT IN WHITE SATIN

As in so many of George's outfits, the emphasis is on layers: the outermost layer is a pure white housecoat or hospital coat. The sleeves have been turned back and buttoned to reveal the cuffs of a white, collarless shirt.

You might find one of these in the wardrobe of an older relative or alternatively you could unpick the stitches and remove the collar of an ordinary white shirt. Between the coat and the shirt, George wears a quilted, sleeveless pinafore. Cotton trousers are worn under the pinafore: you can easily make them or, alternatively, wear white long-johns. The shoes are weird and expensive, but by tying and sticking white ribbon to white training shoes you can achieve a similar effect.

George completes his outfit with two butterfly brooches and a necklace.

In this picture, the rest of the group are dressed in dazzling suits. You can easily achieve this effect by sprinkling handfuls of glitter on an old dinner suit.

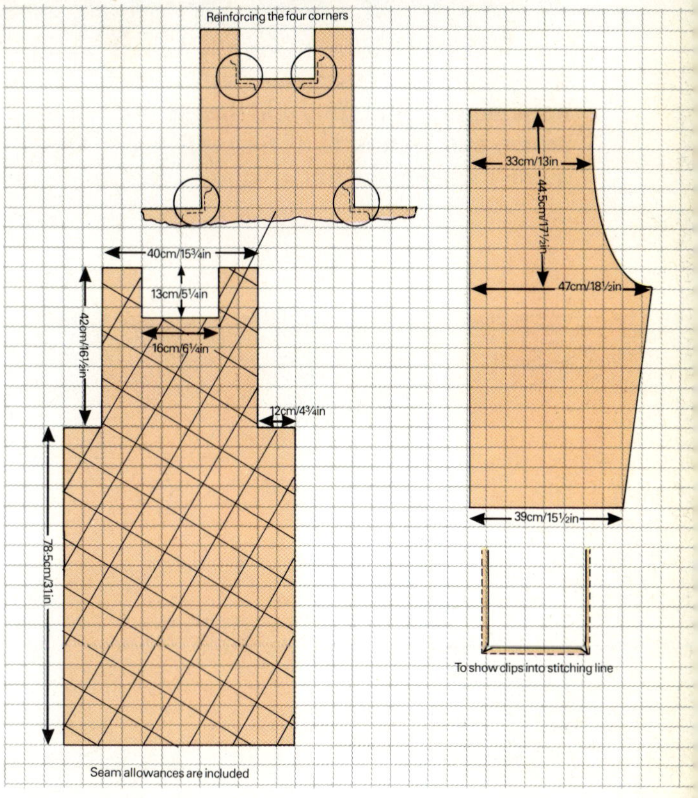

Pinafore and trousers
Both these patterns are very simple to make – the pinafore is made from just two straight-angled pieces, plus a facing, and the trousers have an elasticated waist.

Materials
For the pinafore:
2.5m/2⅔yd of 90cm/36in-wide light-weight quilted fabric or plain medium-weight white cotton fabric.
1 reel of white thread.
For the trousers:
2.5m/2⅔yd of 90cm/36in-wide medium-weight white cotton fabric.
1 reel of white thread.
1m/1yd of 2.5cm/1in-wide elastic.

Making the pinafore
Use the measurements given with the diagram to make a pattern (measurements include 4cm/1½in for the hem and 1.5cm/⅝in on all other seams), and cut two. Make a facing pattern and cut two facings.

On each of the four pieces, reinforce the four corners by stitching on the seamline as shown in the diagram.

Join the main pieces at the shoulder and side seams then do the same with the facings.

With right sides together, join the facing to the neck edge, then clip up to the stitching line at the corners and turn the facing to the inside.

Clip up to the line of stitching at the armhole corners on the facing and main body. Turn under the seam allowances and tack then slipstitch the facing to the armholes. You can trim back the seam allowance on the facing by about 5mm/¼in if the effect is too bulky.

Put the pinafore on to check the length, cutting a strip off the bottom if necessary, then make the hem.

The trouser pattern
Make a pattern using the measurements given and bending a wire coat hanger to help you to draw the curve. Measure from crutch to just above ankle bone for inside leg measurement. The side seam will be this measurement plus 44.5cm/17½in.

If your waist is larger than 77cm/30in, add 5cm/2in to each measurement apart from side and inside leg seams, which remain the same.

Sewing the trousers
Using the pattern, cut four pieces (two pairs). Take two matching pieces (to make a leg) and join the side seam and the inside leg, then do the same with the remaining two pieces. Join the legs together round the curve.

Turn under 1.5cm/⅝in and then 3.5cm/1⅜in at the waist and hem round (you can use your machine and stitch right through), leaving a 3cm/1in gap.

Measure your waist, take 9cm/3¾in off this measurement and cut elastic to this length (for example, if your waist measures 79cm/31in, you will need 70cm/28in of elastic). Thread the elastic through the channel made by the hem and then secure the ends together with a few strong stitches.

Check the length at the ankles, trimming if necessary, and hem (4cm/1½in hem) as normal.

HOT HATS

Boy George's hats are, literally, his crowning glory. Each and every one has so much individuality that they add that special punch and glamor to all his outfits. They are quick to make and fun to wear.

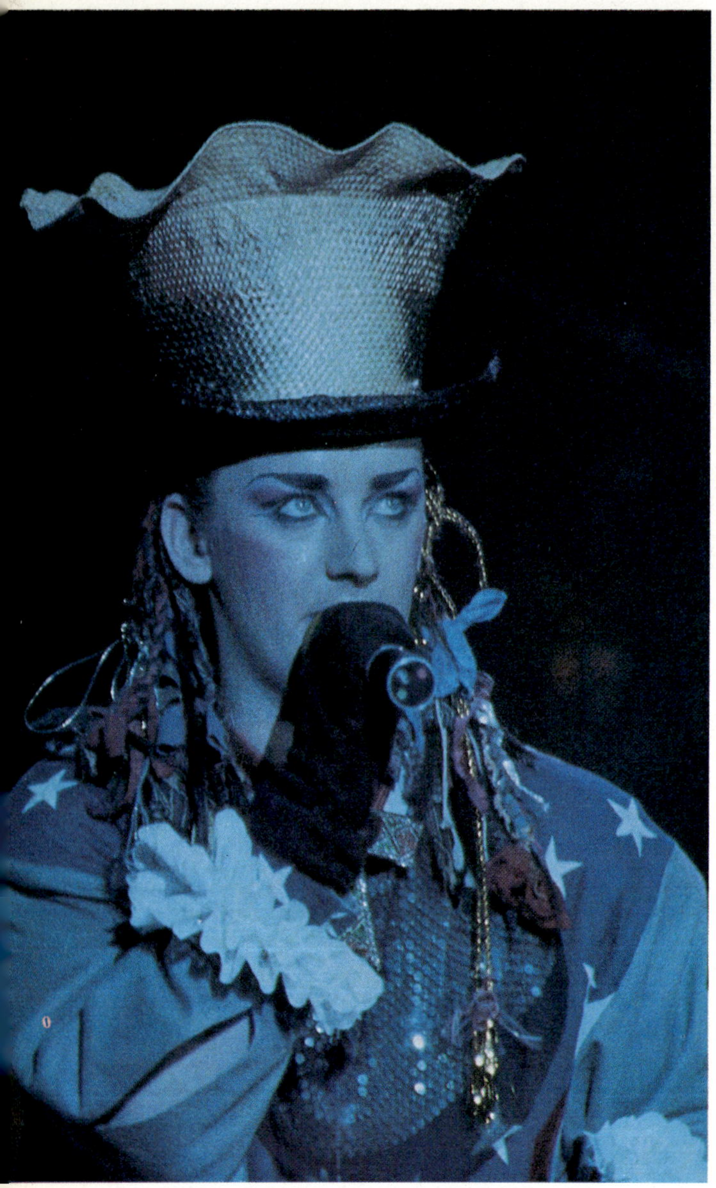

The Mad Hatter
The first of the hats shown here is loosely based on that worn by the Mad Hatter in *Alice in Wonderland.*

Materials
Wicker waste paper basket (old or new, in a fine weave).
Straw hat.
Glue or button thread.
Fabric paints.

Making the hat
Cut the bottom from the basket and make slits, as shown, all round the rim and the lower edge. Make the slits about 7cm/2¾in deep (*Fig 1*).

Next, hold the basket over a steaming kettle of water until the rim of the basket begins to curve outwards where the slits have been cut. Be very careful when doing this to keep your hands well away from the steam. The steaming should give you the petal shape at the top of the hat.

Repeat the procedure with the bottom edge of the basket, creating a similar effect to the top.

The basket can now be placed over the crown of the straw hat and stuck down with glue or stitched on by hand, using strong thread (*Fig 2*).

The final stage is to paint the hat, either as seen in the picture or in colors of your own choosing.

A simpler version of the hat would be to buy an old top hat from a secondhand shop or cadge one from an older relative, then cut the top off and fray the edges, before painting it with fabric paints.

Fig 1

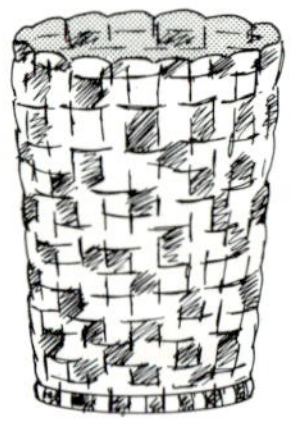

Slits –

Fig 2

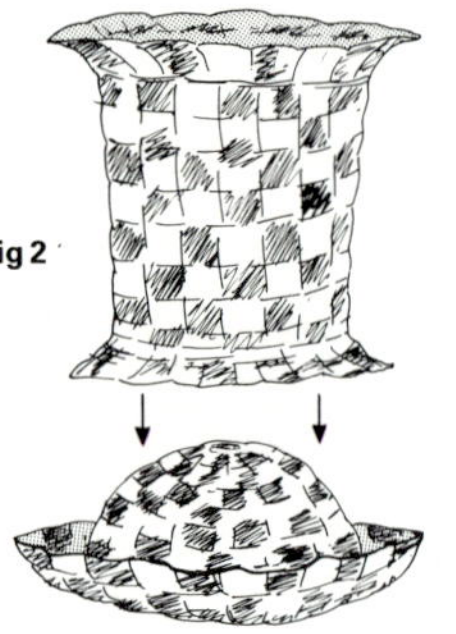

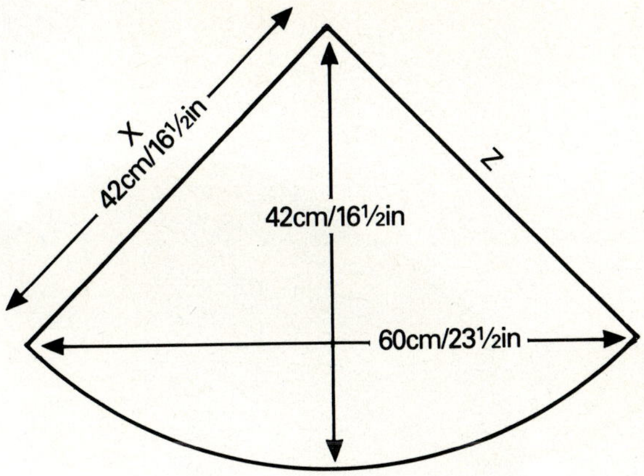

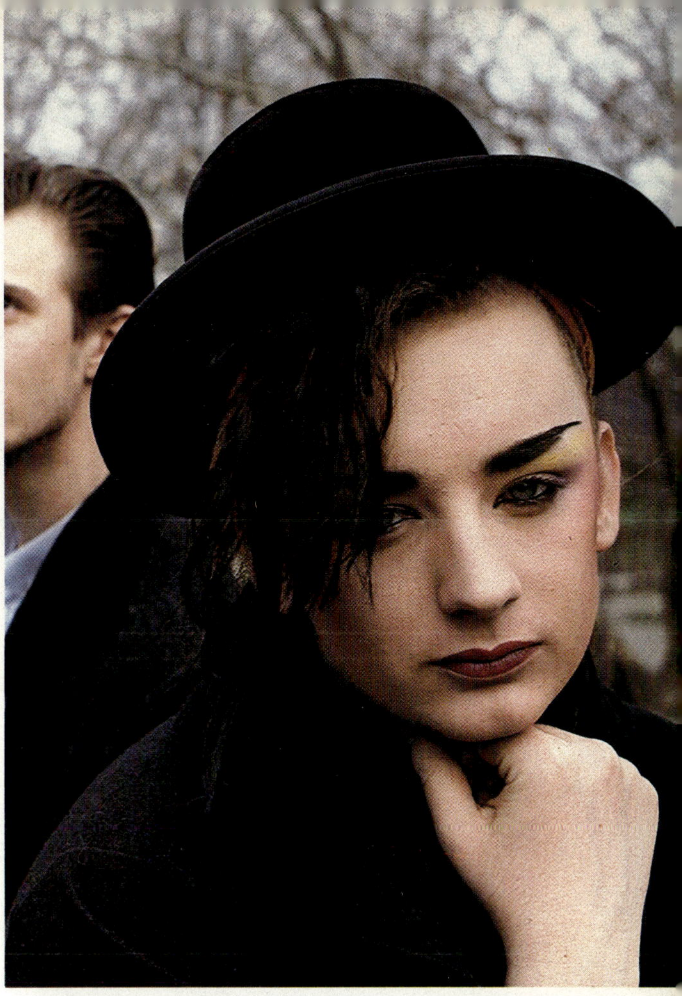

Sequinned hat (*see page 14*)
George's extravagant hat looks expensive but in fact it is easy to make one very similar.

Materials
Stiff card.
Sequins.
Net or lace (you can have a mixture of different nets and laces).
Thread to match.

Making the hat
Draw the shape according to the dimensions given in the diagram and cut out.

Join edges X and Z, using either staples or sticky tape.

Cover the resulting funnel with the fabrics and trimmings until there is no card to be seen, securing the fabric to the hat with a few stitches. Leave an overlap of fabric at the opening of the hat so that you can wrap it round your head to hold it in position.

Silver hat (*see page 12*)
This is another quick-and-easy but very dramatic hat. Simply take an ordinary straw hat and dye it with gold or silver spray paint.

Trilby
A pushed out trilby is one of Boy George's favorite hats and can be created in a matter of seconds. Take a conventional trilby hat, push the top outwards with your hand then curl the edges of the brim slightly upwards. You can easily add a bright colored ribbon to replace the existing hat band. This hat can be worn with almost any Boy George outfit.

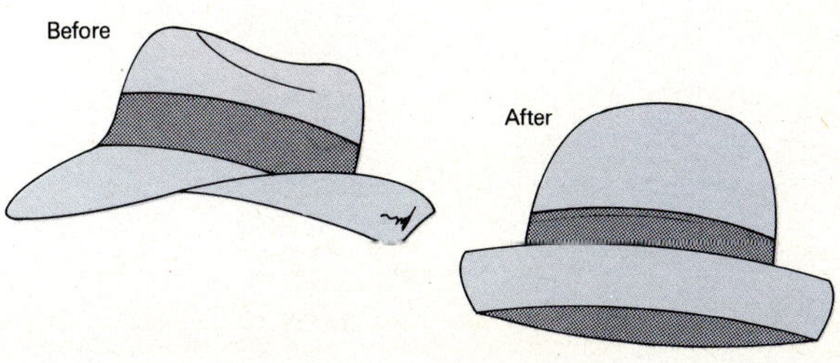

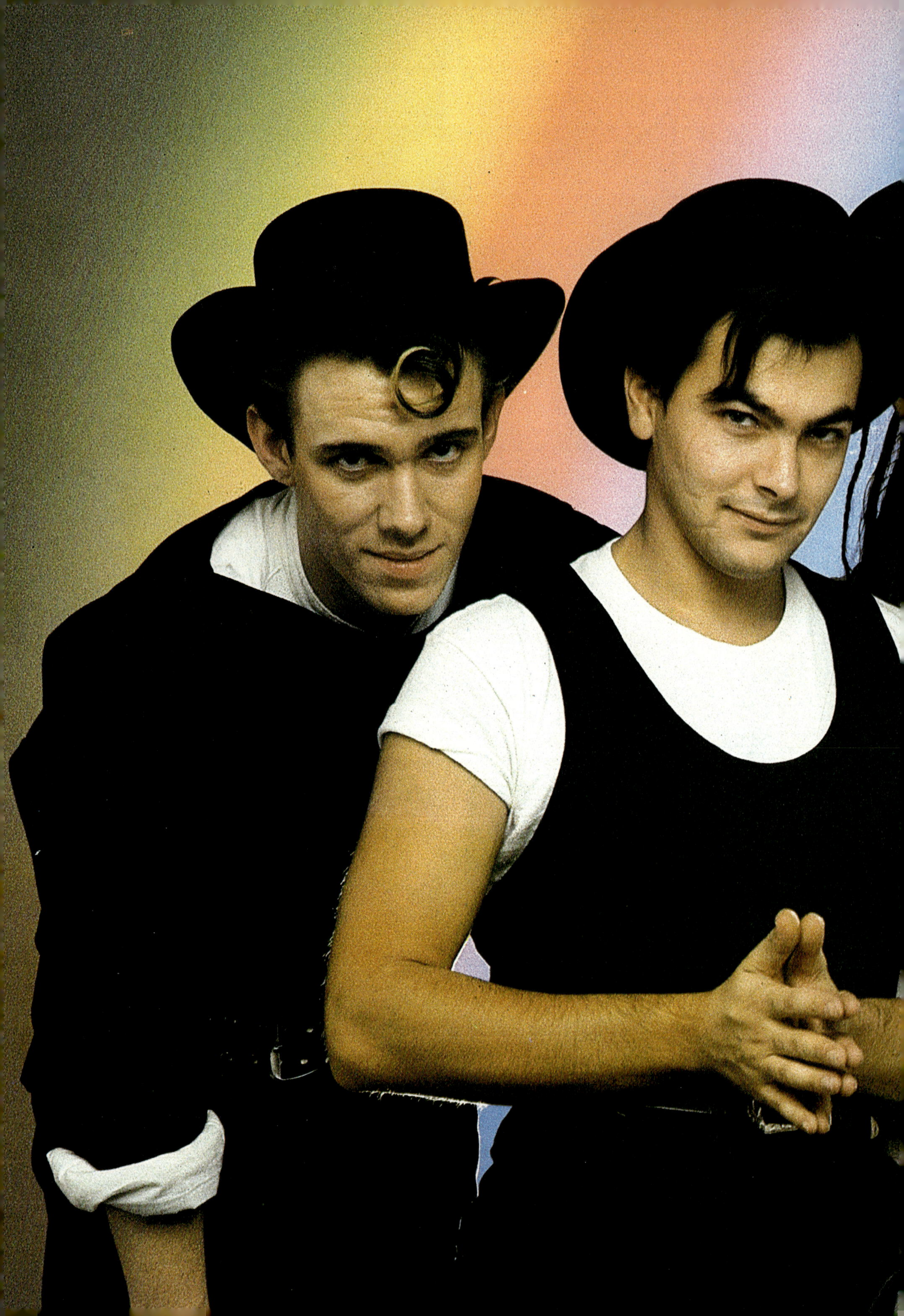

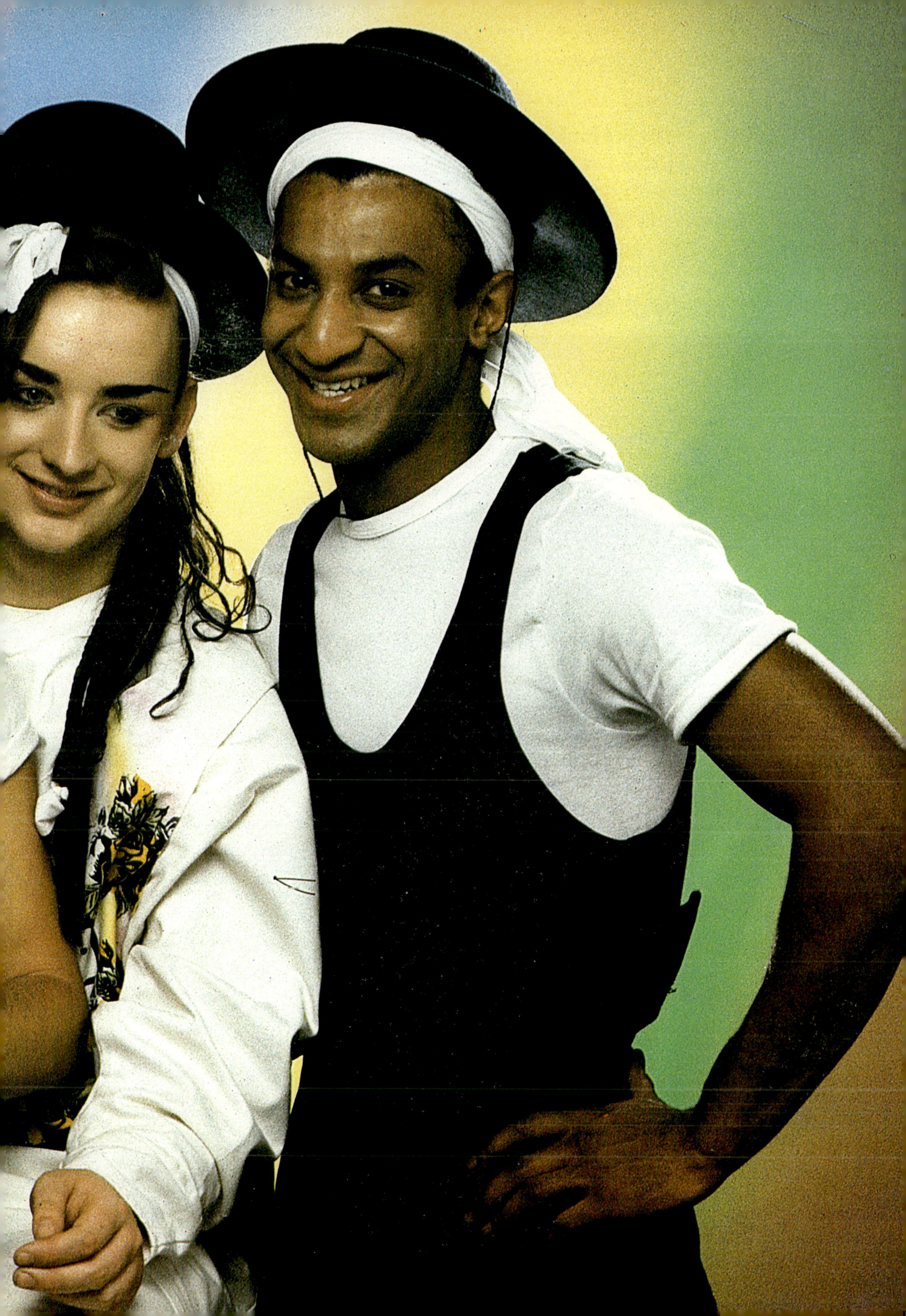

“A lot of people think I look pretty excessive, but I think I’m pretty normal. I love wearing make-up. I like to wear lots of colors and give myself a real bird of paradise look.”

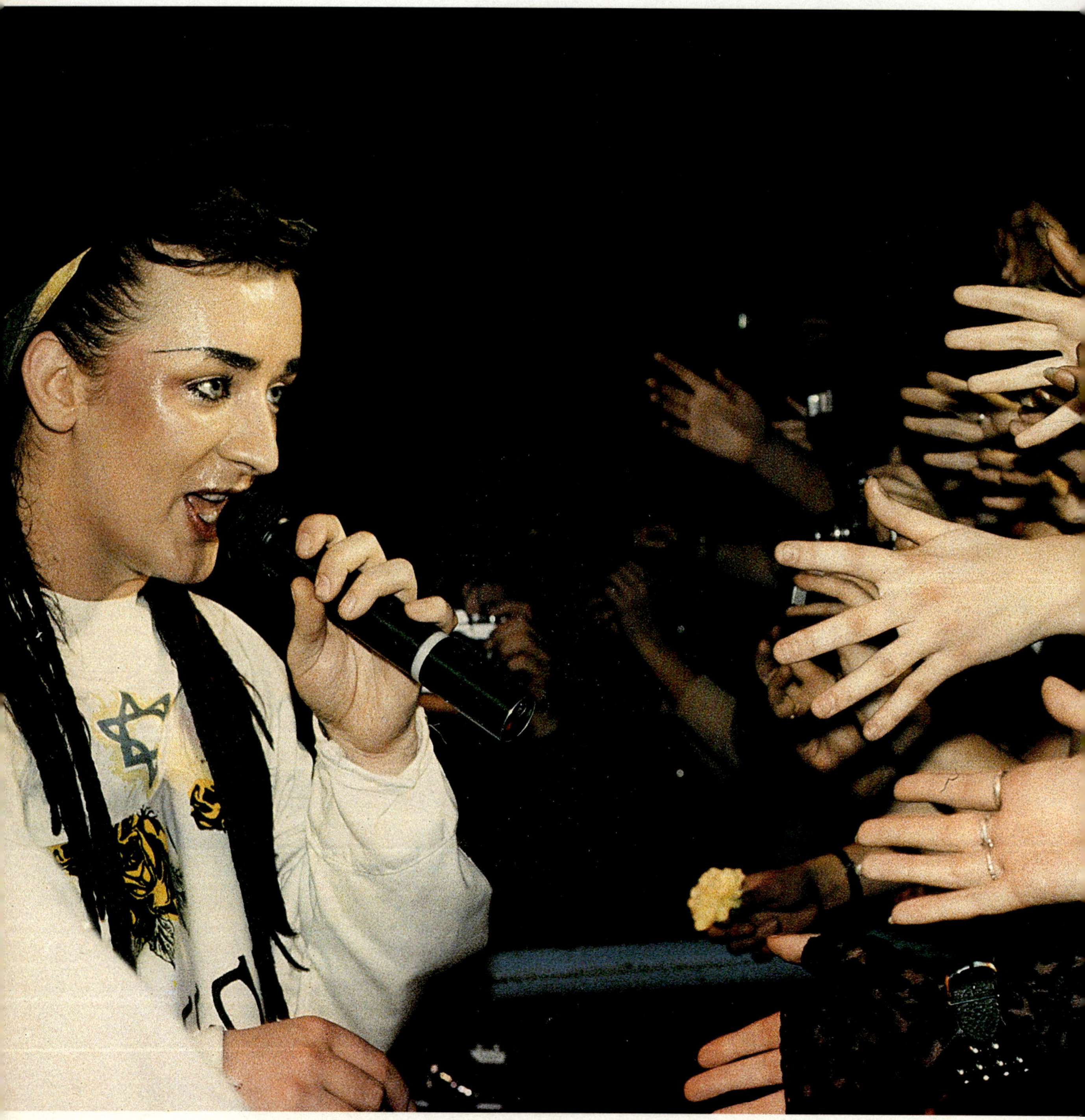

MAKE-UP HINTS

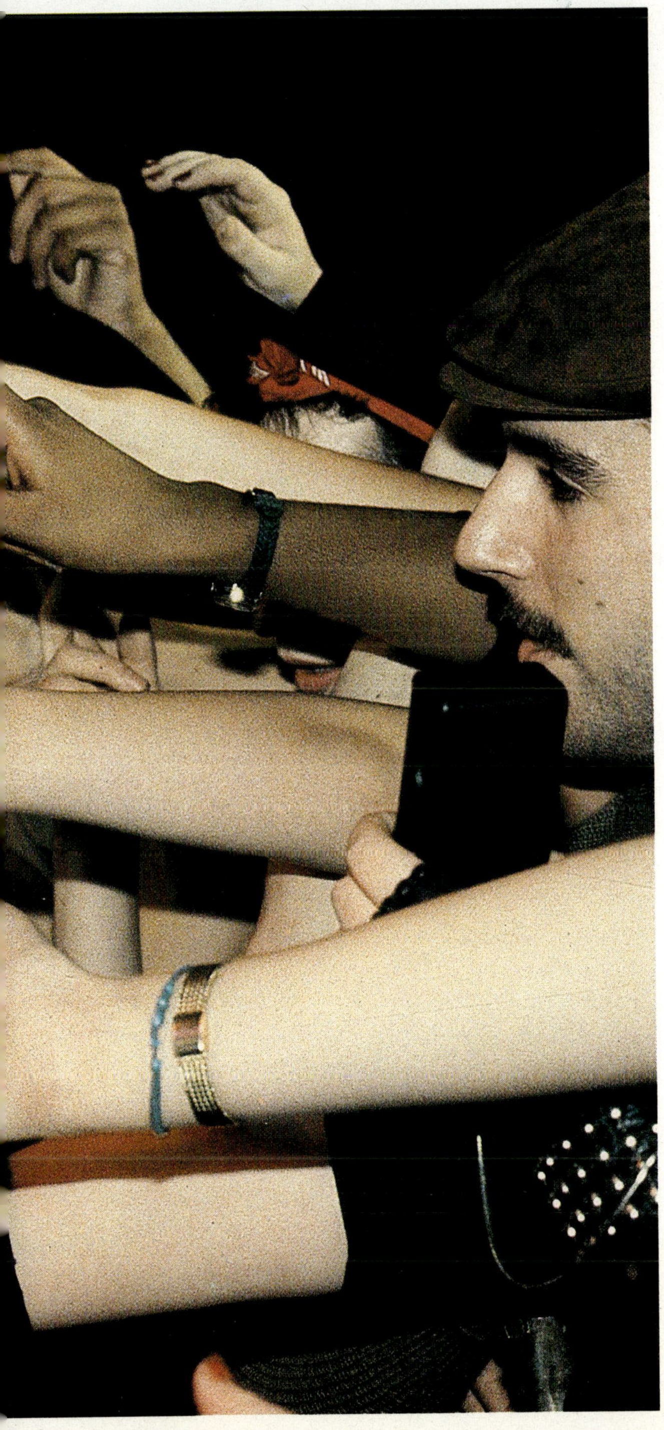

Moisturizers
It is a good idea to prepare your face before starting to apply any make-up. Moisturize it, using any product which suits your skin type. *Creams* tend to be heavier than *lotions* and so are better for dry skin.

Concealers
If you have circles under your eyes or any spots or blemishes, cover them with a light *concealer* or *cover-up cream*. Concealers need to be blended in and brushes do the job extremely well.

Foundations
These come in *liquid*, *cream*, *stick* or *cake* form. The liquids are the lightest, gently coating the skin, and generally do not provide enough color for Boy George faces.

Creams are thicker, can be applied with fingertips or sponge and give a shiny appearance.

Sticks are thicker still, can be applied directly and then blended in with fingertips.

Cakes add a lot of color but will dry the face. Best suited to oily skin types. They need to be applied swiftly with a damp sponge to avoid the possibility of streaking.

Cleansers
For removing make-up, use a *cream* or *liquid* cleanser. Soap and water will dry the skin too much. Of the types available, creams are best for dry skins since they tend to cling to the face. Massage onto the face and remove with a tissue. Cold creams and liquids suit all skin types and are again applied with the fingers and removed with tissues.

There are also water-based cleansers which can be washed off, while others come on wads of absorbent fabric. The cloth-impregnated ones are particularly good for smaller areas, such as around the eyes.

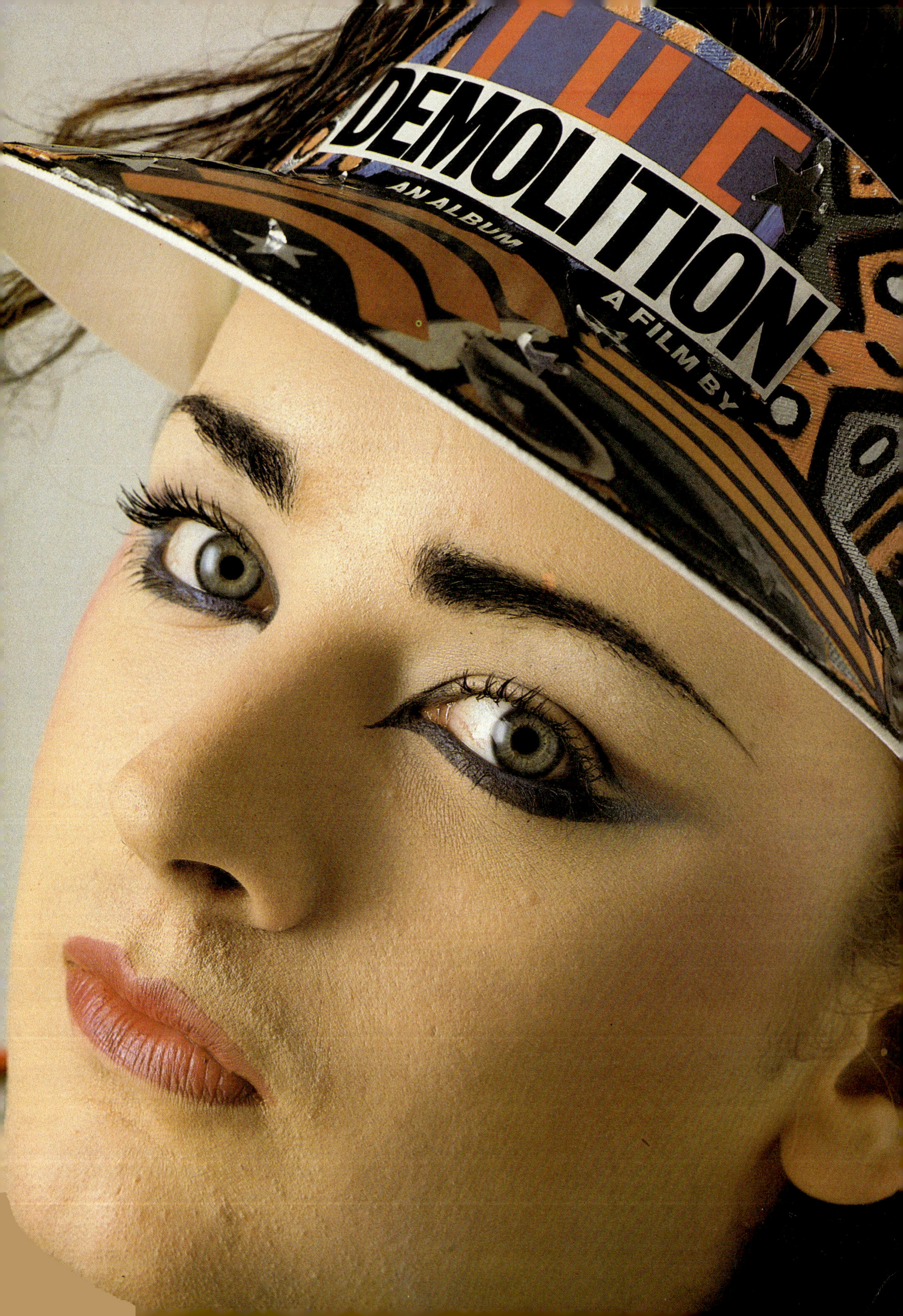
DEMOLITION
AN ALBUM
A FILM BY

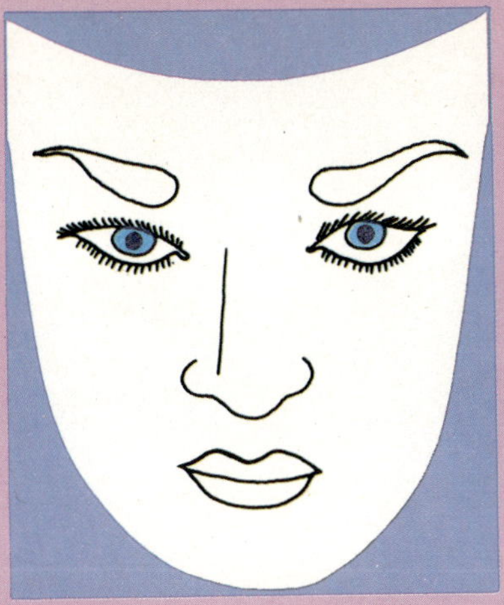

Foundation/Powder: To achieve a pale face use either a very pale or white panstick or white pancake.

Panstick is oil-based and can be applied with fingers or a damp sponge. It needs to be thoroughly powdered with a light or white powder (baby talc can be used). Press the powder on well using a powder pad, then brush off excess with large powder brush.

Pancake is water-based and leaves a matt finish. It should be applied with a damp sponge in short swift strokes. It dries very quickly and can streak if not applied speedily.

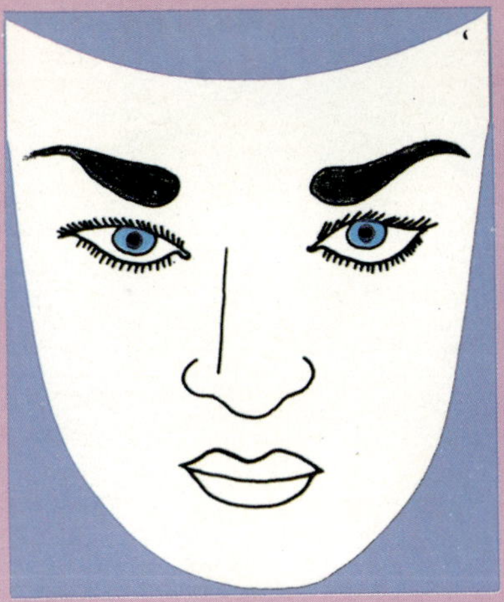

Eyebrows: The brows here are strong and dark. Use either liquid or block eye-liner applied with a fine brush, black powder shadow applied with a hard fine brush, or simply a sharp black pencil.

Black pencil: starting at the inner edge of the brow and making short sharp strokes shape the brow, fading at outer edge. Then powder over the brow and press on well.

Eye-liner: with a fine brush make short sharp strokes simulating hair. Let the liner dry and then continue until you get the desired shape.

Black powder: this is a good method for someone who already has dark brows. A chisel-shaped brush is best.

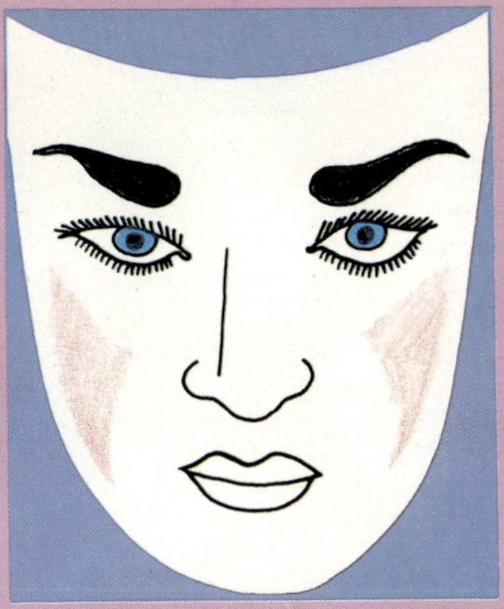

Blusher: Apply pink blusher on the pad of the cheek using a big blusher brush. Always tap or blow off excess powder on brush before applying blusher. Remember that you can easily add more blusher but it is messy to remove it if you put on too much. Build up gradually. Powder over edges to blend.

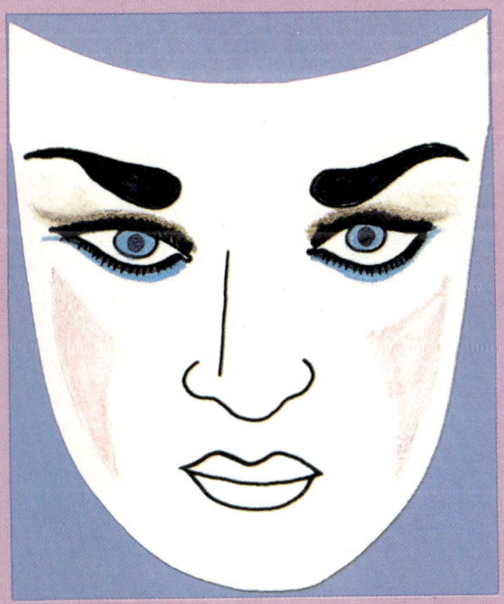

Eyes 1: Using a dark brown shadow and an eye-shadow brush, apply powder to socket area, starting at inner corner of lid and taking the line straight out. Always tap or blow off excess powder shadow before applying to skin.

Using blue eye-liner or a blue pencil, draw in stylized line under eye, fading upwards and outwards at outer corner. Remember that pencil is greasy and needs to be powdered to set the color.

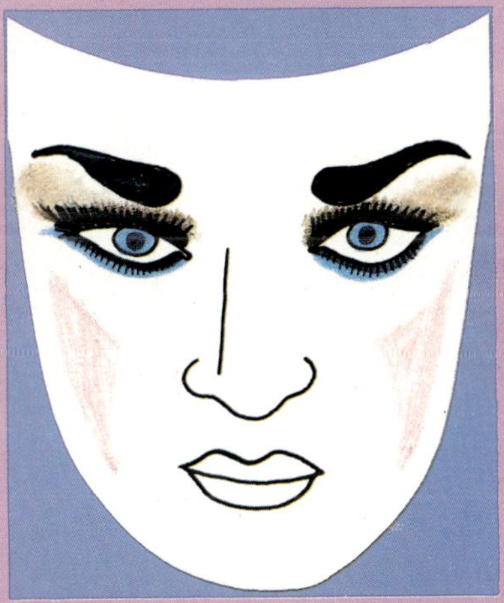

Eyes 2: Apply white shiny shadow to lid and brow bone, slightly overlapping the brown socket line. Apply black mascara (two coats) to top and bottom lashes, allowing first coat to dry completely. Comb lashes through to separate before applying second coat. If lashes are soft, apply face powder between coats to build lashes up.

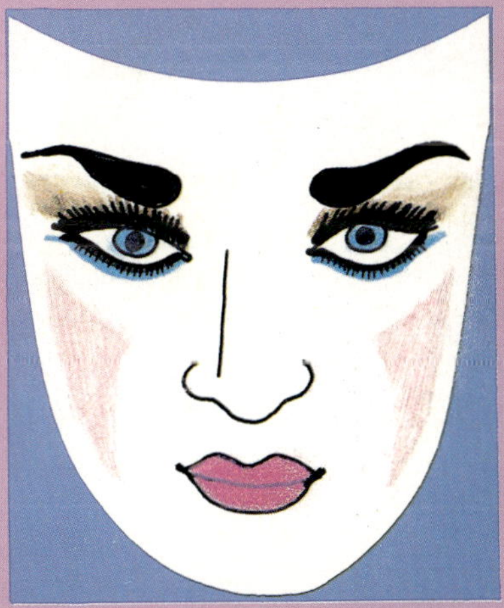

Lips: Dark pink is used here. It can be applied directly but a lip-brush is more accurate. Blot and powder lips. As with eyebrows, the powder serves to set the color and prevent smudging. Pale powder or even baby talc will do. Then re-apply lipstick for longer-lasting effect.

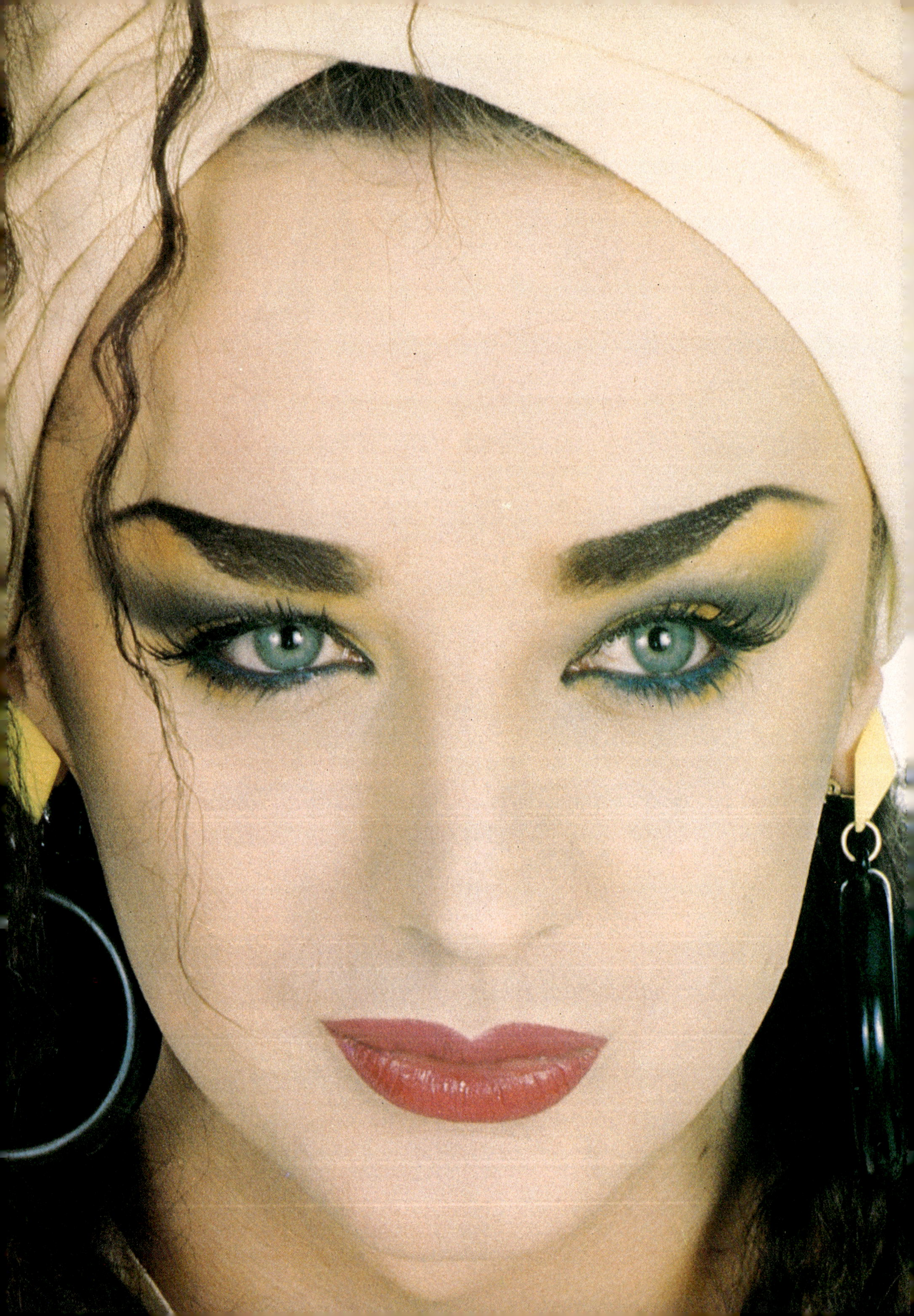

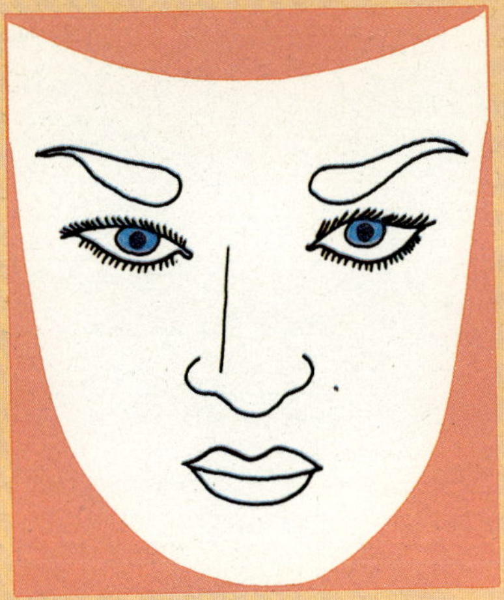

Foundation/Powder: To achieve the soft, but overall white base, use either panstick or pancake make-up. The latter is applied with a moistened sponge over the entire face and neck area. *Note:* apply pancake speedily to avoid streaking.

More foundation may be needed for the neck area if skin is a different texture to that on the face. Conceal shadows *before* application of pancake using an ivory tone camouflage stick. A light powder or baby powder will give the face sheen, as pancake is very matt. Apply powder with soft brush.

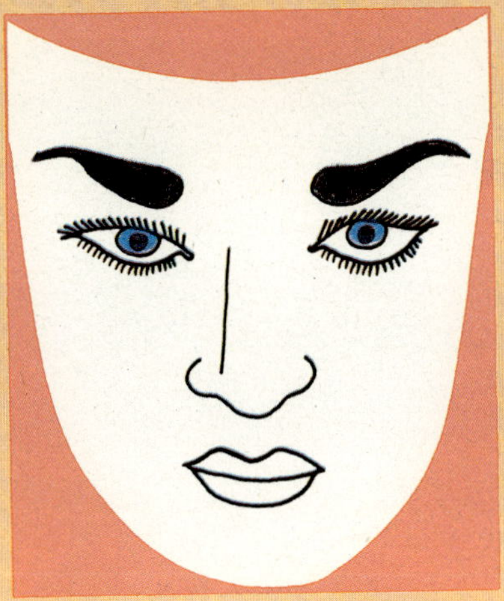

Eyebrows: Using a fine, hard eyebrow pencil in black, and starting roughly in line with sides of the nose at its narrowest, apply a thin line of pencil building up to a hard arch and fading outwards. Always start lightly and build up pencil application. When the correct shape is achieved, powder lightly and repeat action, filling in eyebrows to a sharp, well-defined line.

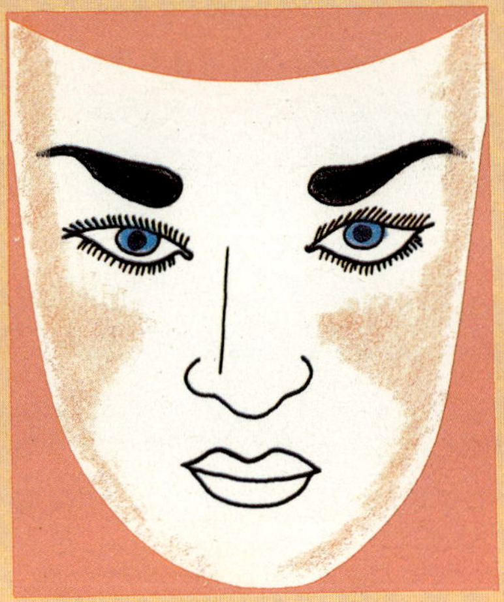

Blusher: Using an orange-red powder blush, dust lightly high above the temples staying close to the hair-line to contour the face. Apply the same blusher over cheek-bones and into hollow. Apply several light coats of blusher.

Blush below jaw line to give a well-defined shape to the face. A mixture of pink and orange blusher gives an interesting effect and more impact.

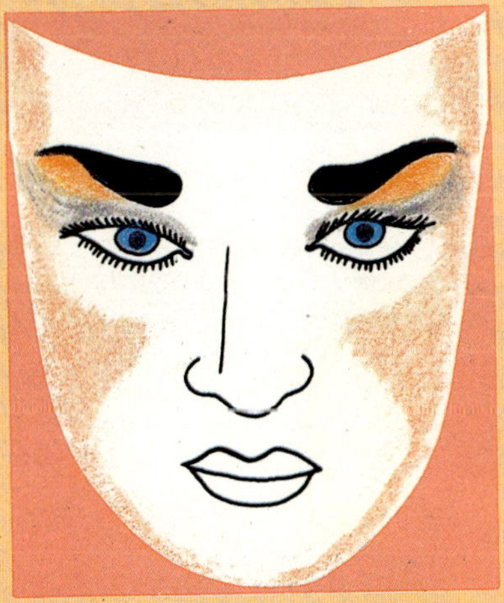

Eyes 1: Charcoal powder shadow is applied to the socket area using a small brush. The shadow starts under the inner brow and sweeps upwards and outwards to almost join outer end of the brow. Take care to blend areas above the socket line. As with the eyebrow, it is better to build up color slowly and gradually. Over the brow bone, add a touch of orange blusher.

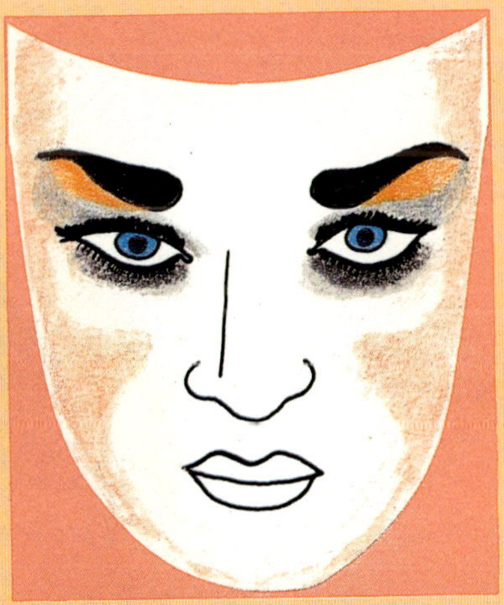

Eyes 2: On top of lid area, apply a shimmery white powder shadow, taking care not to smudge the grey area above. Now, using a sharp, black eye pencil, line the whole eye, staying close to the lashes. Smudge line under the eye with cotton bud to soften. Mascara is applied in two coats to the top and bottom lashes.

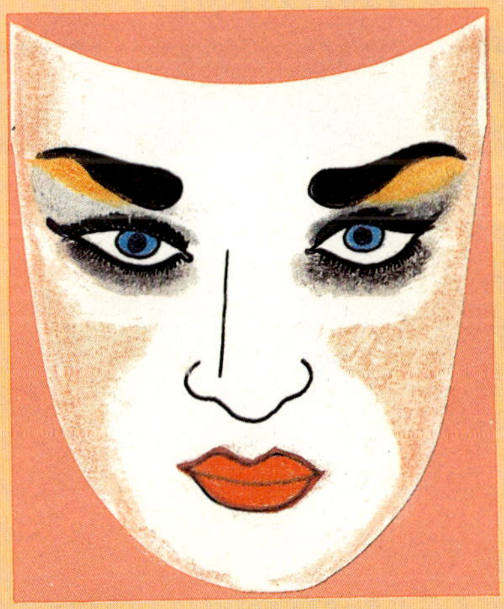

Lips: Using a red lip pencil, outline lips and then fill in with pillar box red lipstick with a brush. Blot with tissue, powder well and repeat action. Make sure that you use a rather hard lip pencil for best results.

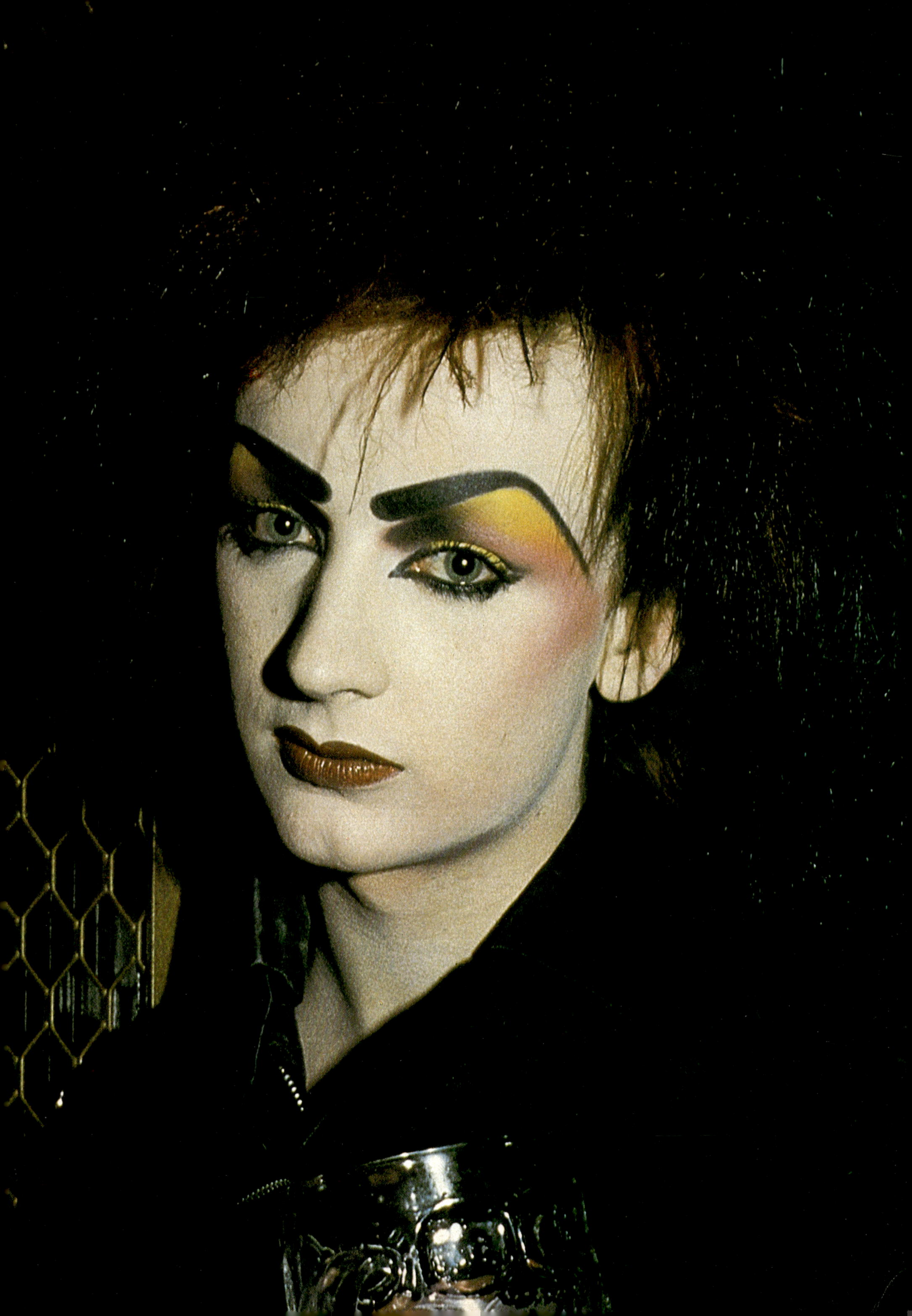

My mother still won't kiss me directly on the lips. She can't cope with the fact that I might put lipstick on her.

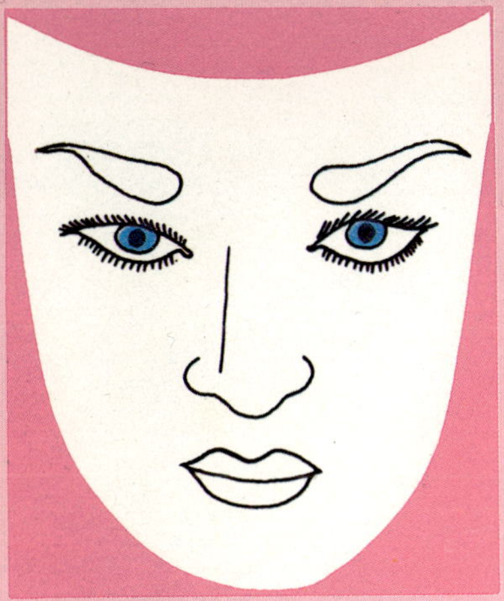

Foundation/Powder: The foundation is actually white here rather than simply pale, giving a more ghostlike effect. Again, sticks or powders can be used (*see page 41*). Any blemishes or shadows under the eyes should be concealed with a good cover-up cream *before* applying the foundation.

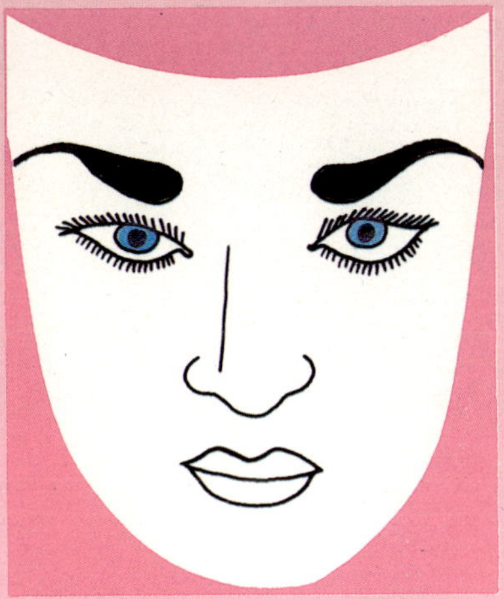

Eyebrows: Using eye-liner and brush, paint in large exaggerated eyebrows. Do it slowly, a little at a time, building up the shape as you go. It is thickest at the inner corner, tapering downwards almost as far as the ear.

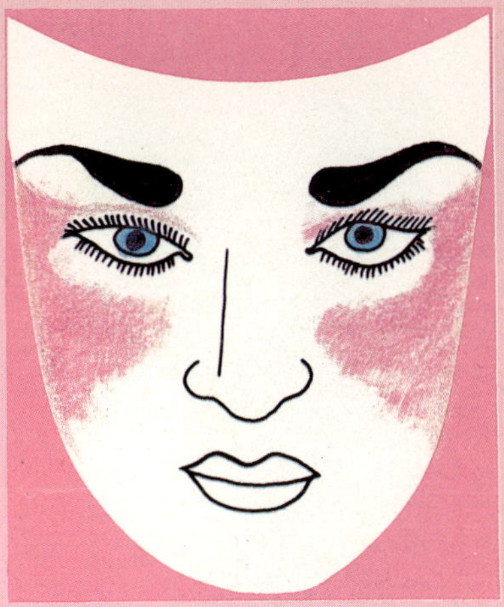

Blusher: Apply pink shadow or blusher to outer eye area. Take it down onto the cheek, letting it gradually fade away.

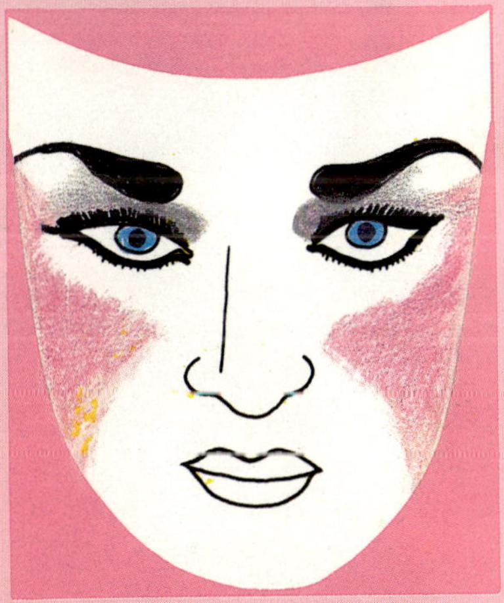

Eyes 1: Outline eyes with black pencil or black eye-liner. Remember that the pencil is greasy and needs to be powdered over. Follow eye shape exaggerating inner and outer corners. Line inner eye with black pencil or kohl.

Using dark grey shadow place a smudge under brow at inner corner, blending it into the pink shadow. If using a brush, don't forget to tap or blow off excess powder before placing the brush on skin or powder will go all over the place.

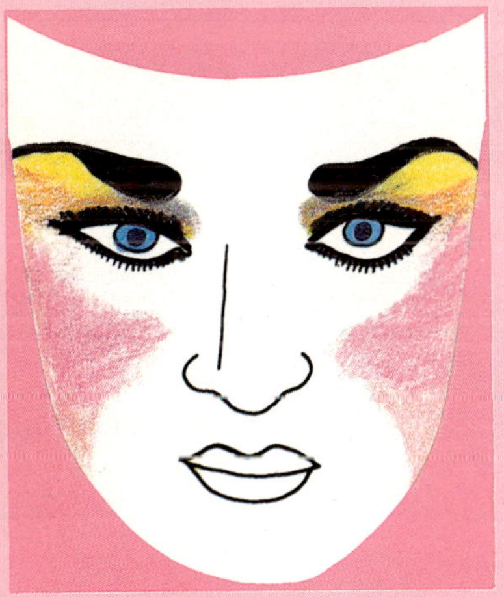

Eyes 2: Apply yellow shadow to lid and brow bone. Make it strong, like a sun-burst, also blending it into the pink blusher.

Mascara top and bottom lashes. When dry, comb through to separate lashes. Apply second coat.

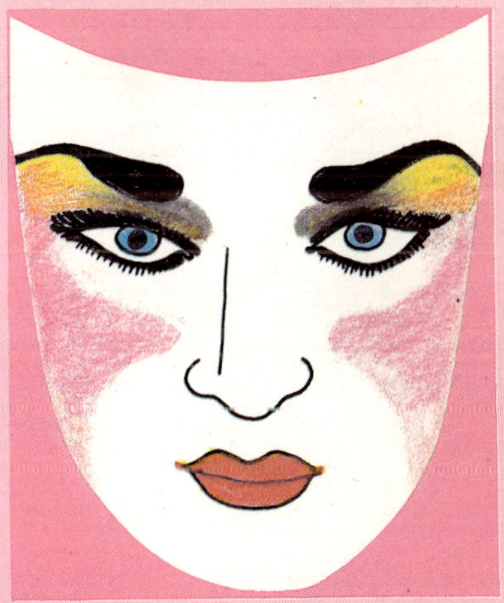

Lips: Outline lips with dark red pencil, blot and powder. Using a brush, fill in lips with dark red lipstick.

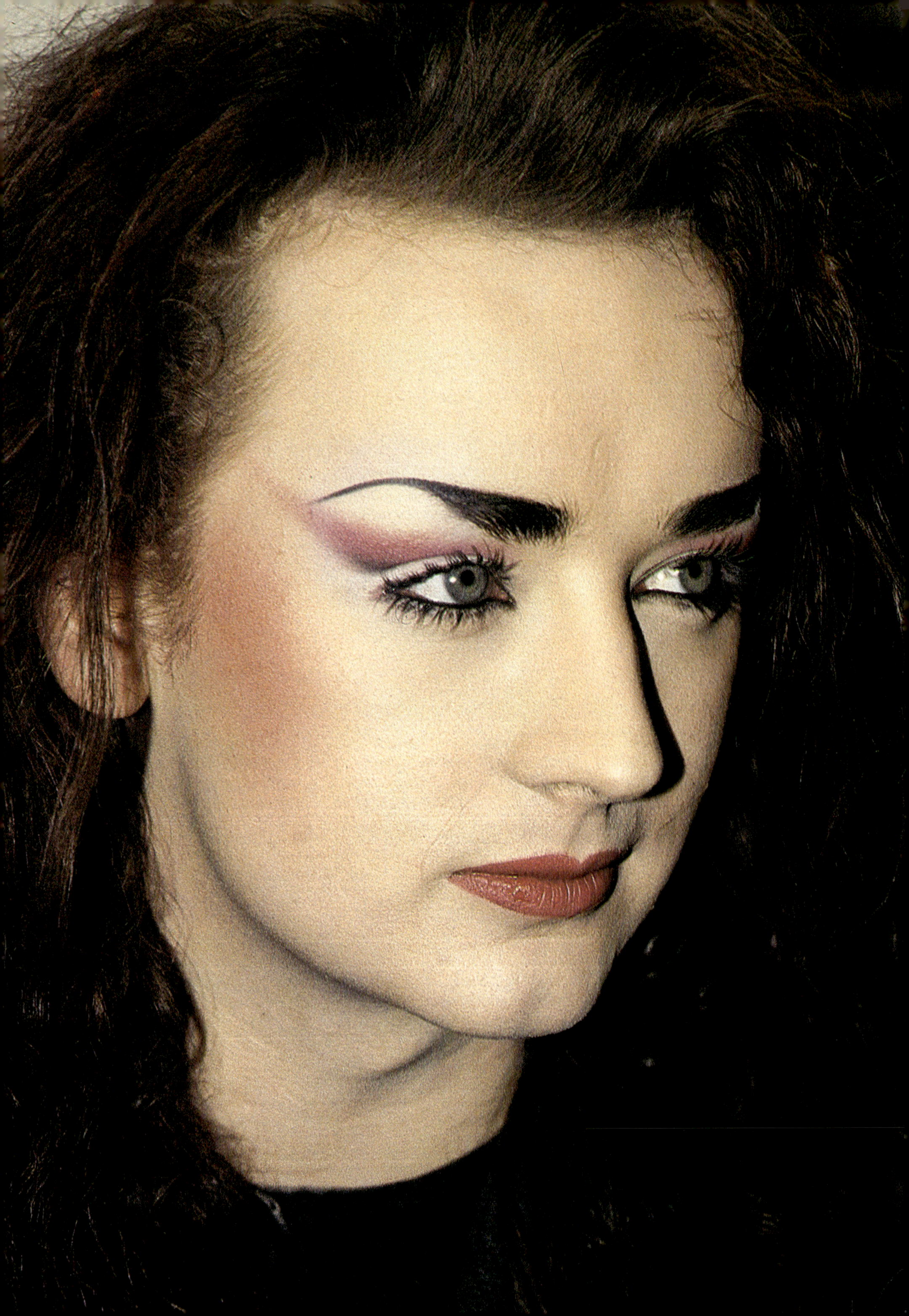

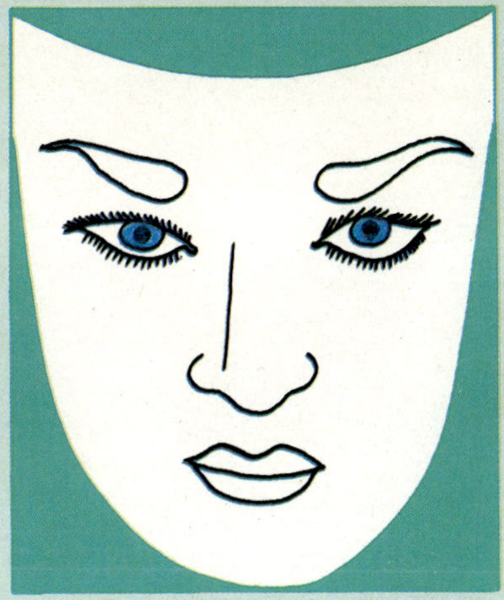

Foundation/Powder: A very pale powder forms the basis of most of Boy George's faces. If you use a panstick, powder it well and apply with a sponge or fingers. Caked powder dries quickly and so needs to be applied swiftly using a damp sponge. For a more complete effect, do the neck as well as face.

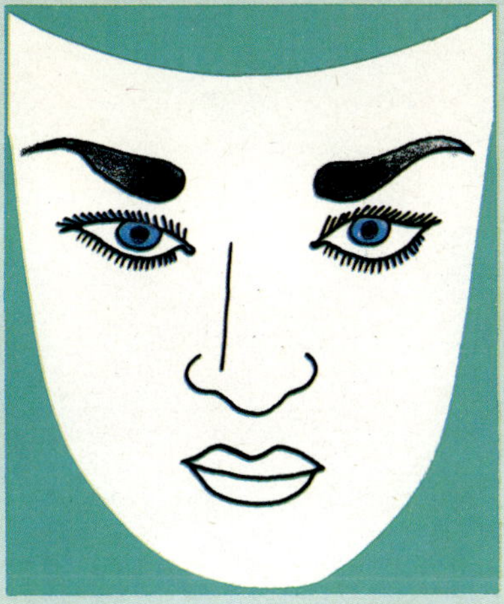

Eyebrows: A fine, hard, black eye-pencil has been used and applied heavily from the inner corner to the arch, fading to a thinner line than that on *page 40*. The exaggerated depth of color gives a more dramatic look.

Once again, powder between applications to prevent color running if skin gets hot under disco lights or through excess activity. The best pencil to use is one that has a built-in sharpener at the end. Otherwise, sharpen pencil with a razor to a flat, wedge-shaped point, and apply with the fine side.

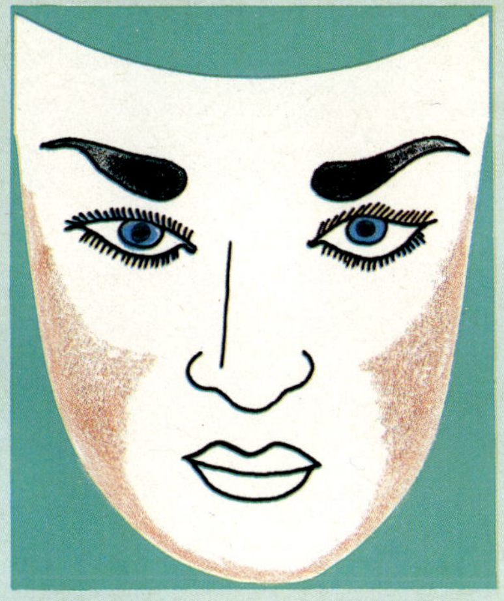

Blusher: Powder blusher in deep russett is lavishly applied this time to hollow areas below the cheekbones only, to give a strong, well-defined look. Make sure a matt shadow is used as shimmery blushers have a tendency to "flare" under lights, or give a silver foil effect. Blush under jaw line, but don't be heavy-handed.

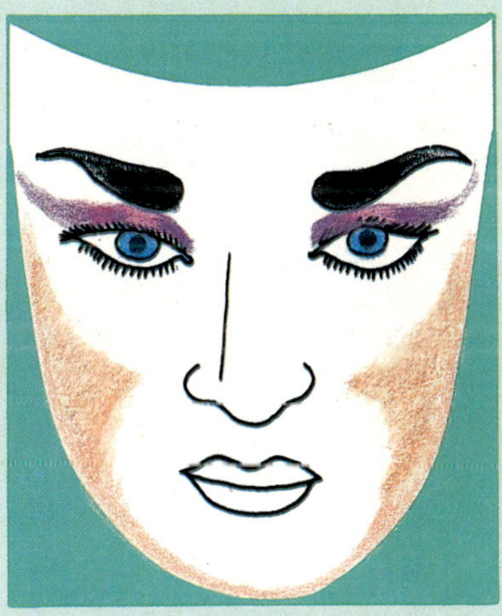

Eyes 1: Following socket line, start at the inner corner of the eye and extend shadow outwards and upwards, carrying line beyond the outer corner of the eyebrow. The shadow should be heavier away from the centre of the lid and fading to the outer point. Here, a deep purple tone has been used. Take care to blend above the socket line area.

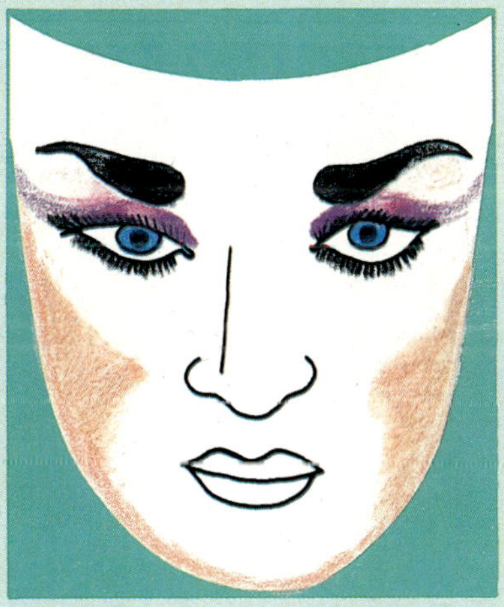

Eyes 2: Over the lid, dust shimmer ivory powder shadow, going no further than the outer corner of the eye. With a fine liner brush, draw lines on upper lid close to the base of the lashes, widening at the centre and out. Under eye, smudge black kohl pencil.

On brow bone, dust white frosted shadow to light up the eyes. Apply lavish coats of waterproof cream mascara to top and bottom lashes.

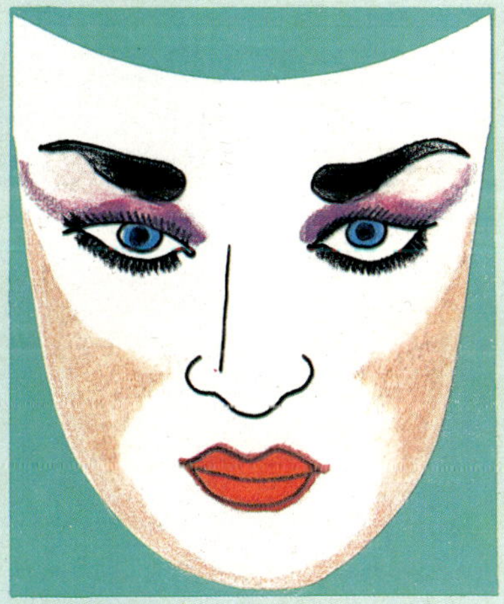

Lips: These are outlined with deep crimson lip pencil. Fill in lips with brick-red lipstick, using a flat lip brush. Blot with tissue, dust on loose powder with powder brush and re-apply colour. The dusting over of powder ensures lips will not "bleed" at the edges.

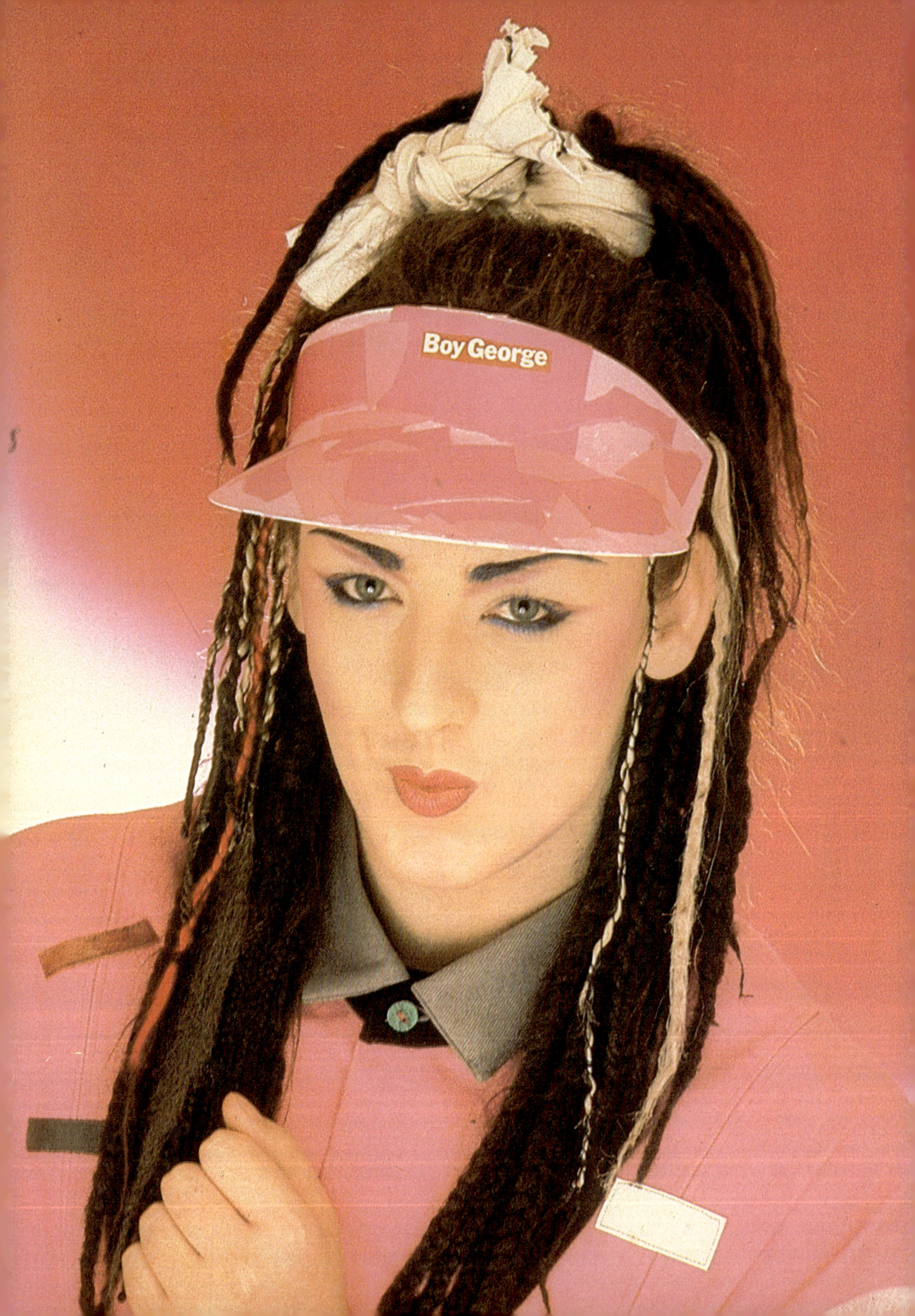
Boy George

"People see that I wear make-up and look effeminate. But I don't think I'm an effeminate or feminine person at all really. I've met lots of people far worse than I am."

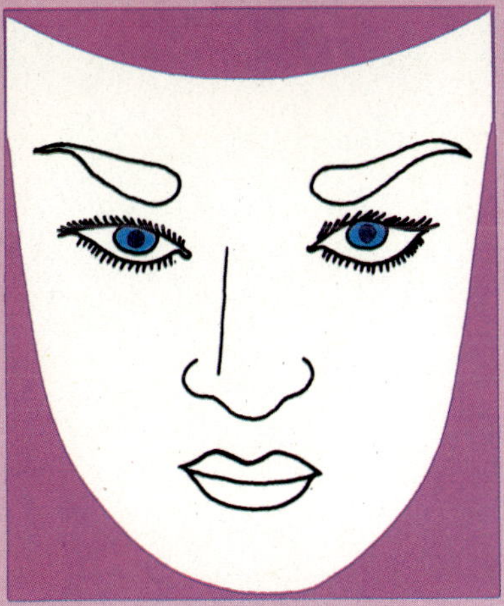

Foundation/Powder: After moisturizing your skin, conceal any blemishes with a cover-up cream, blending it carefully into the surrounding areas. You are now ready for a pale foundation which comes in either cream or powder form. The choice is up to you and depends on your skin type and particular preference.

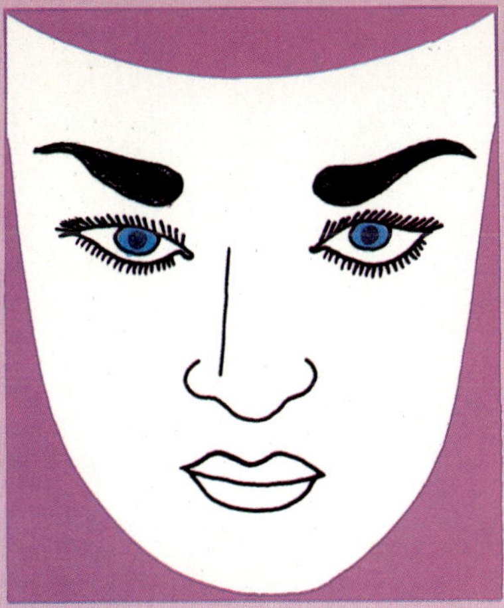

Eyebrows: A black pencil, eye-liner or black powder can all be used to achieve this effect. For different techniques *see page 41*.

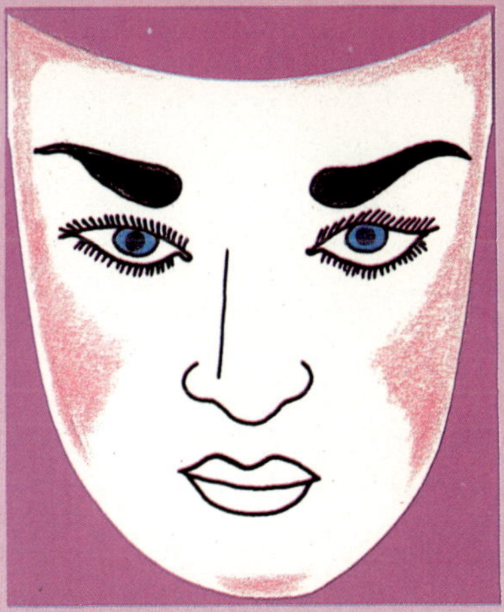

Blusher: Using bright pink blusher and a big blusher brush, apply blusher under cheekbone and blend upwards and outwards to hair line.

Dust a little more on brow and under chin.

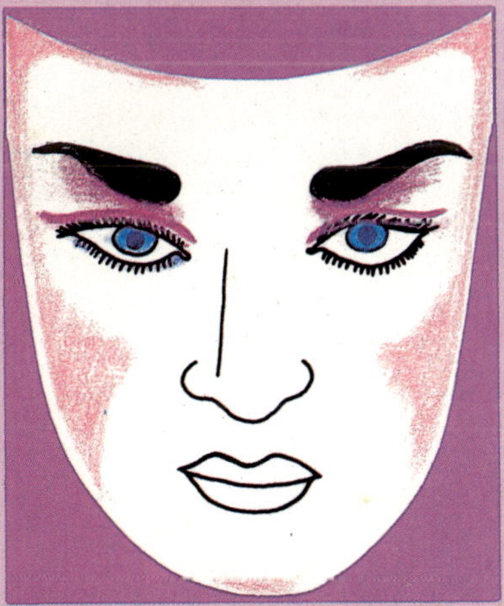

Eyes 1: Using dark pink shadow and shadow brush, draw a thickish line under inner corner of brow fading towards outer corner. Using the same color draw in a finer line from inner corner of socket extending out beyond edge of eye.

Fill in rest of eye area with cream or white shadow to highlight the eyes and brows.

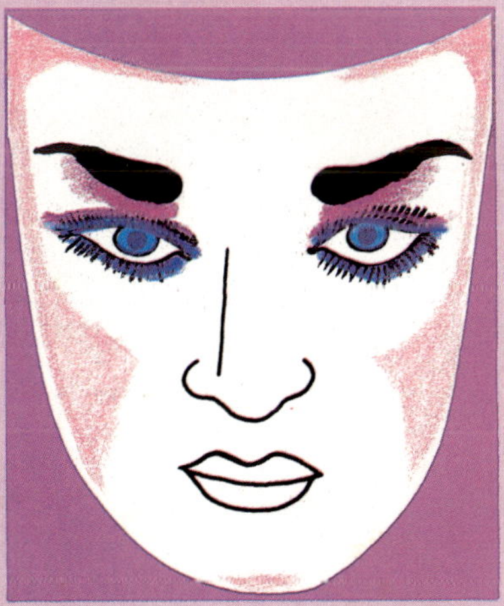

Eyes 2: Using blue eye-liner paint in thickish line under lashes extending this at outer corner. Now paint a very fine line along top lashes to meet bottom line at inner and outer corners of the eyes.

Mascara top and bottom lashes – applying two coats in the normal way.

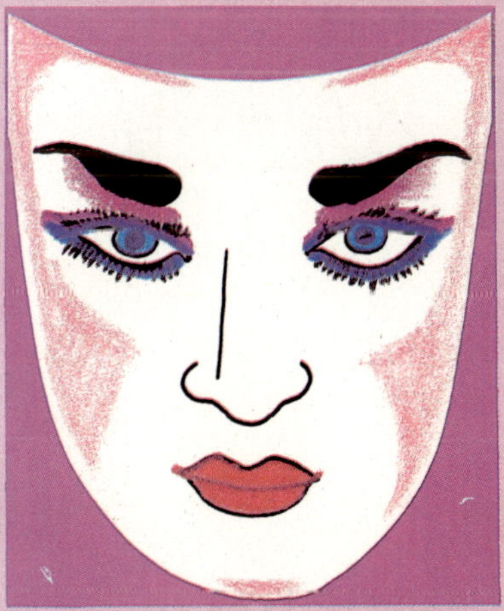

Lips: Outline lips with dark pink pencil, blot and powder. Now fill in lips with same dark lipstick.

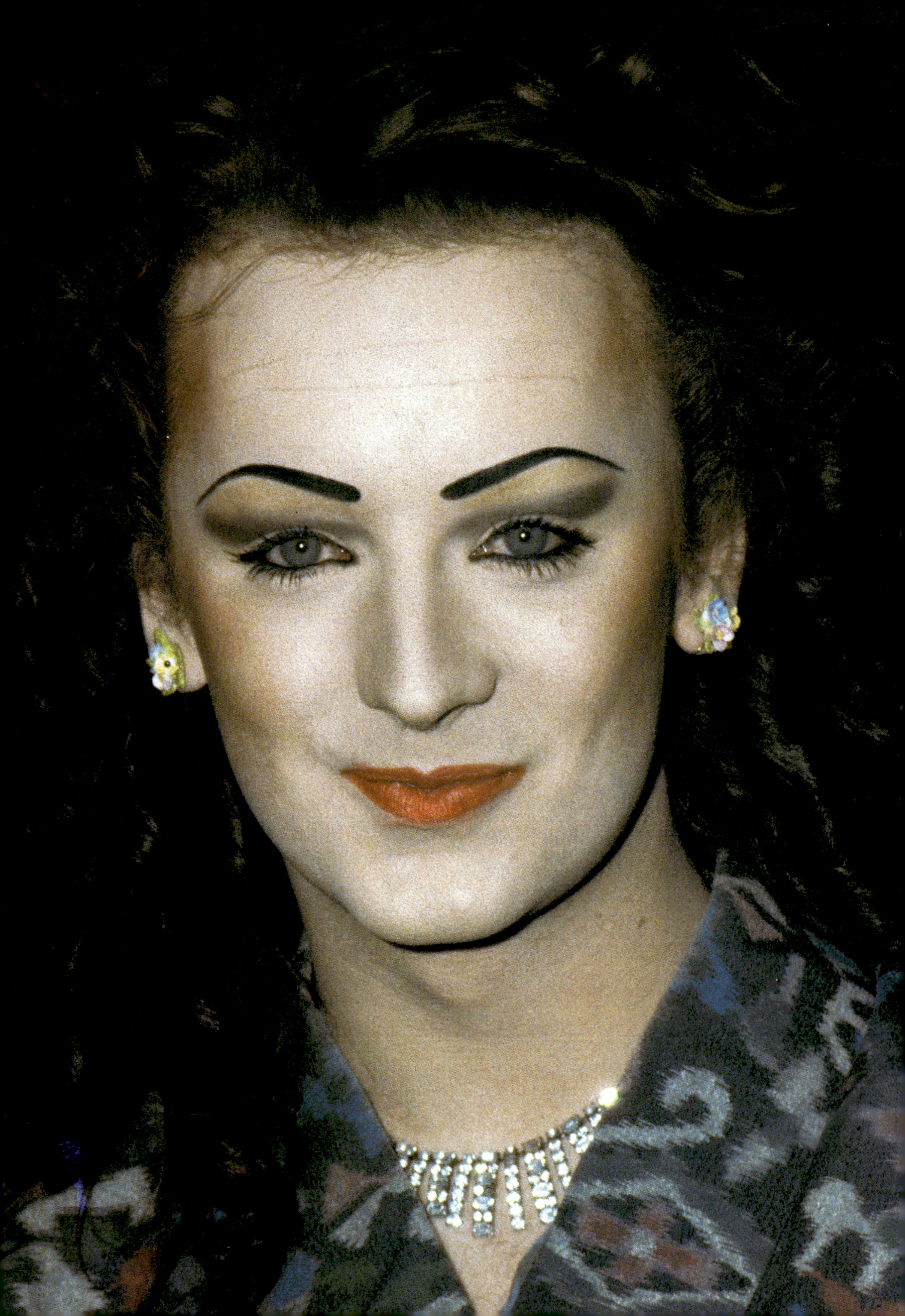

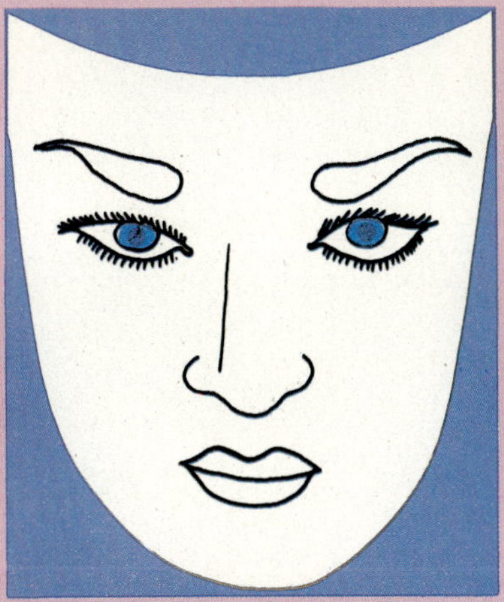

Foundation/Powder: Panstick (a long lasting foundation) should be applied with middle two fingers to a clean face. Take care to apply well to ears, eyelids, eyebrows and neck area. To conceal shadows, apply more panstick with a small brush.

When base is complete, start at the eye area and, using a large velour puff laden with a pinkish-white powder, press into base firmly. Use a lot of powder to cover all shine. Take care over eyelid area. Remove excess with a soft brush.

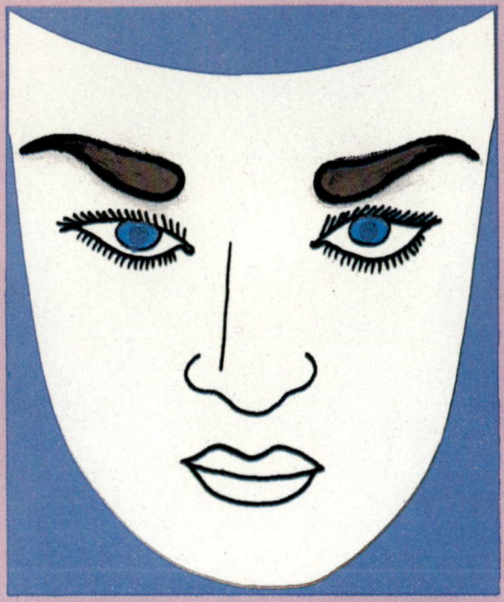

Eyebrows: Using a finely pointed brown eyebrow pencil, fill in the outline using small, feathery strokes. Note that Boy George's eyebrows arch above and parallel to the outer corner of his eyes. Now use a black pencil to provide the final shape, keeping the darker shading towards the outside edges. Two colors allow for heavy but still natural looking eyebrows. (A hard tipped brush can be used to soften lines.)

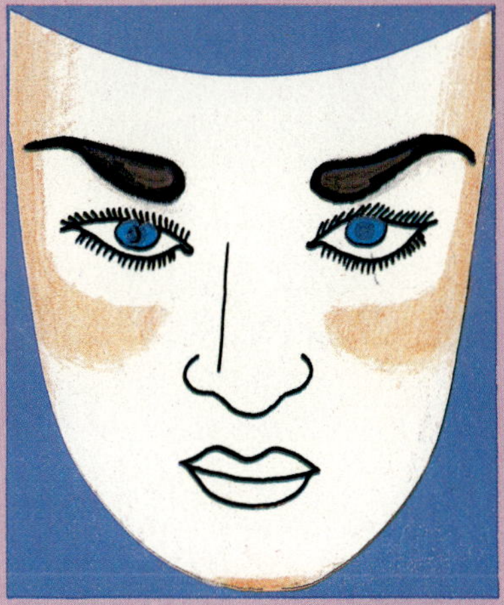

Blusher: Using a tawny blusher and large fluffy brush, apply blush to upper cheek and temple and blend upwards and outwards. With what is left on the brush, touch under chin. Powder edges to blend.

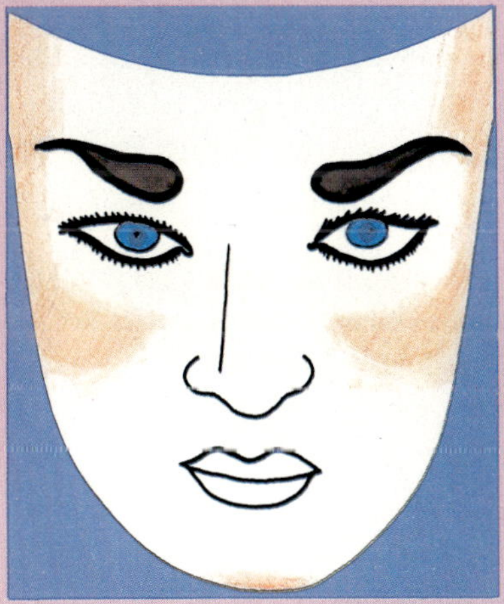

Eyes 1: The eyes and lips are emphasized for this more conventionally glamorous face. Use black eye-liner to outline eyes keeping close to lashes. The line widens slightly at outer corner. Then line inside eye with black pencil or kohl.

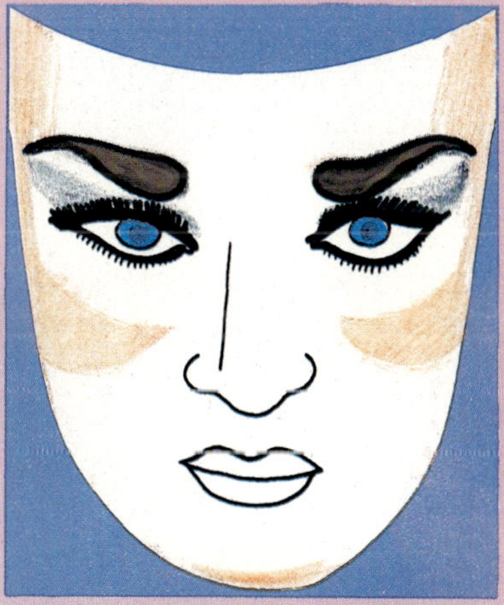

Eyes 2: Using dark grey powder and eye-shadow brush, follow socket of eye from inner corner taking the shadow upwards and outwards at outer corner. Clean the brush and blend grey powder upwards.

Using cream shadow cover brow bone and lid overlapping onto grey.

Apply two coats of mascara as before.

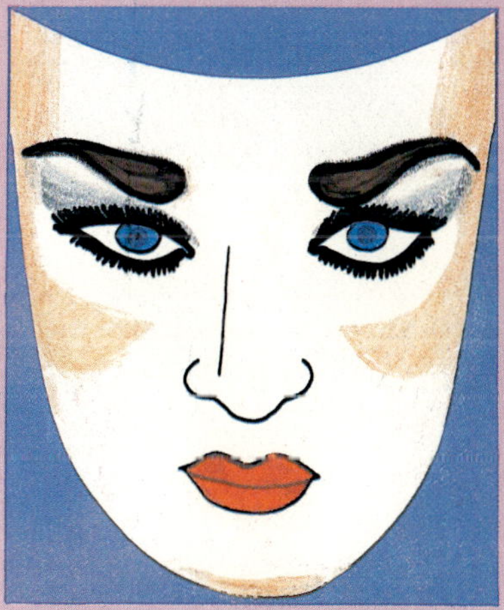

Lips: Apply red lipstick shaping top lip. You may well find it easier to pencil an outline first. Blot lips with tissue, dust on loose powder with powder brush and re-apply color.

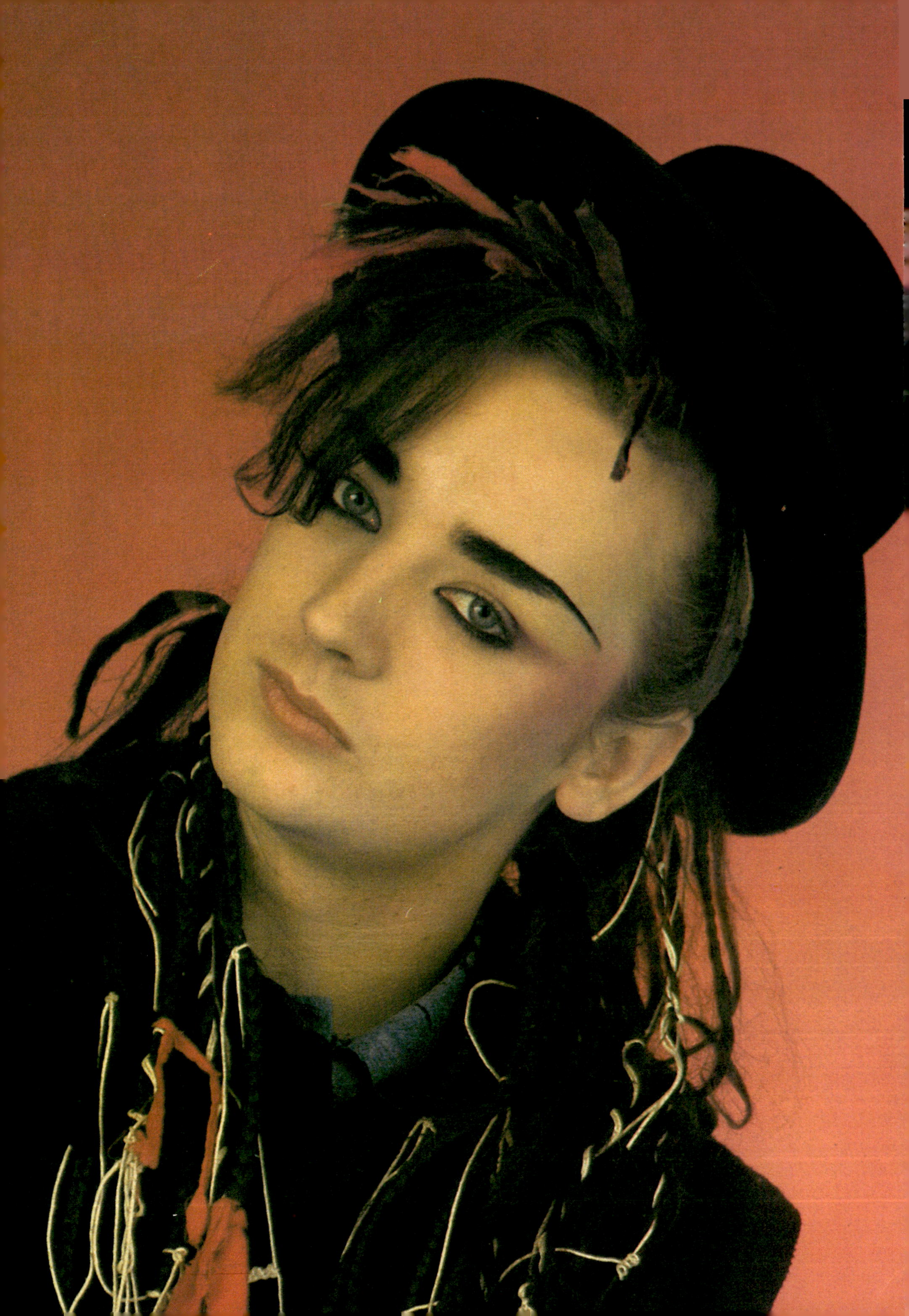

Most people don't want to be different because it frightens them. They've got this fear of alienation. Of not being accepted. It's different with me because I couldn't give a damn really.

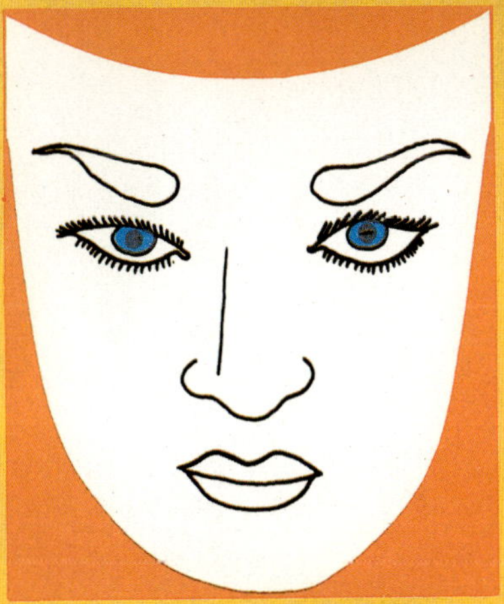

Foundation/Powder: For this dreamier look use ivory panstick, applying it either with fingers or a damp sponge. Powder over carefully, brushing off any excess powder.

Remember to moisturize skin and conceal any shadows or blemishes *before* applying foundation.

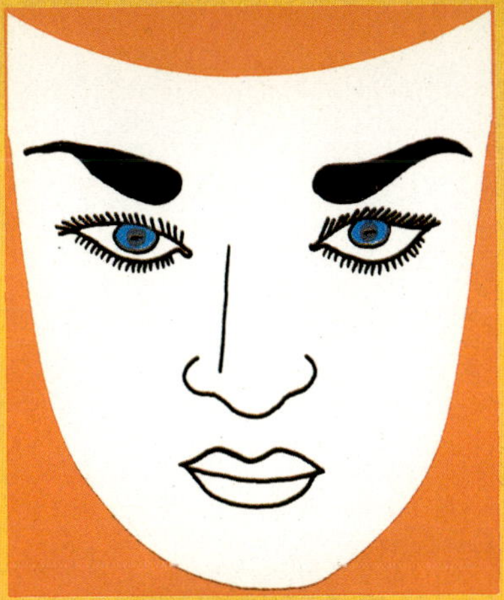

Eyebrows: These are typically strong and dark, but less arched than some of Boy George's faces. To achieve this effect, eye-liner, an eye pencil or black powder can all be used, as explained on *page 41*.

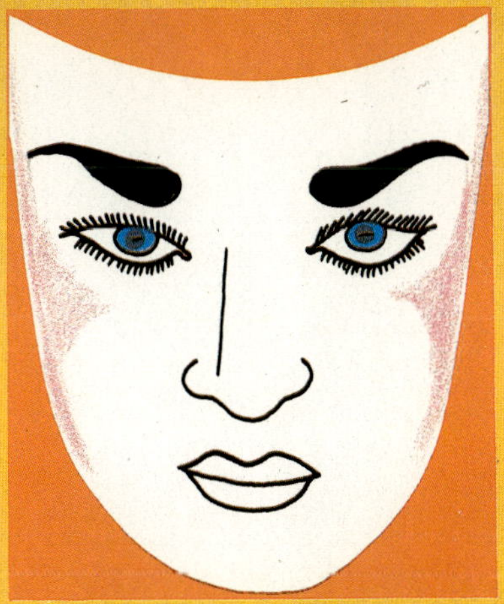

Blusher: Use fuchsia blusher for cheeks and eyes, applying it with a blusher brush.

Place blusher high up above cheeks level with eyes and by means of a round movement, feather blusher onto cheek pad, reaching right back to the hair-line.

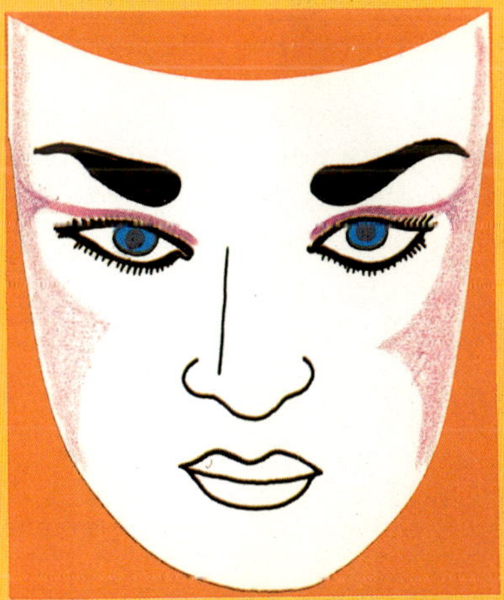

Eyes 1: Relatively little make-up is called for here and so needs to be put on with care. Using a pencil, draw a very fine line above top lashes and a heavier one below bottom lashes. Line inside eyes in black.

Next take fuchsia blusher and eye-shadow brush, and draw in socket line taking color out to meet blusher on cheekbone, and outer corner of the lid.

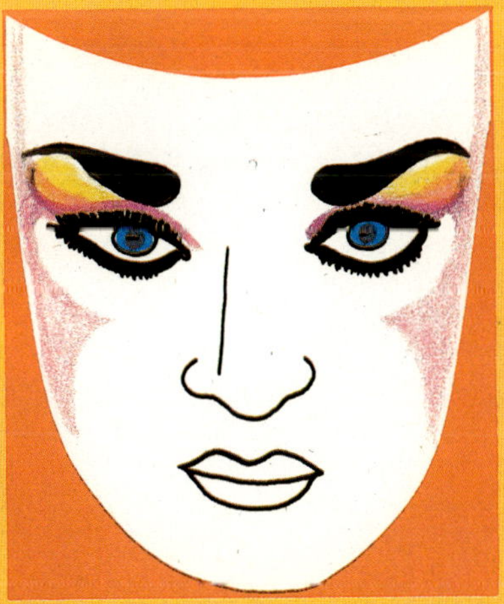

Eyes 2: This look calls for pale yellow shadow blended over the brow bone and inner lid. Fingers or a brush would be fine here. The yellow then meets and blends into the fuchsia.

Mascara top and bottom lashes. Two coats are needed and as usual you should allow the first to dry and comb the lashes through before applying the second coat.

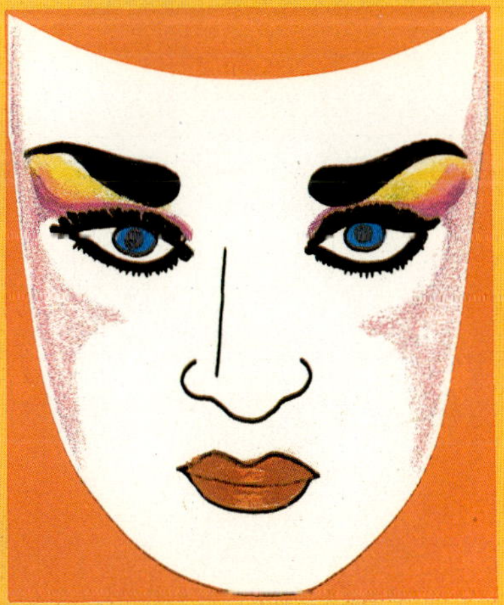

Lips: Using pale tawny lipstick, paint in a soft natural mouth.

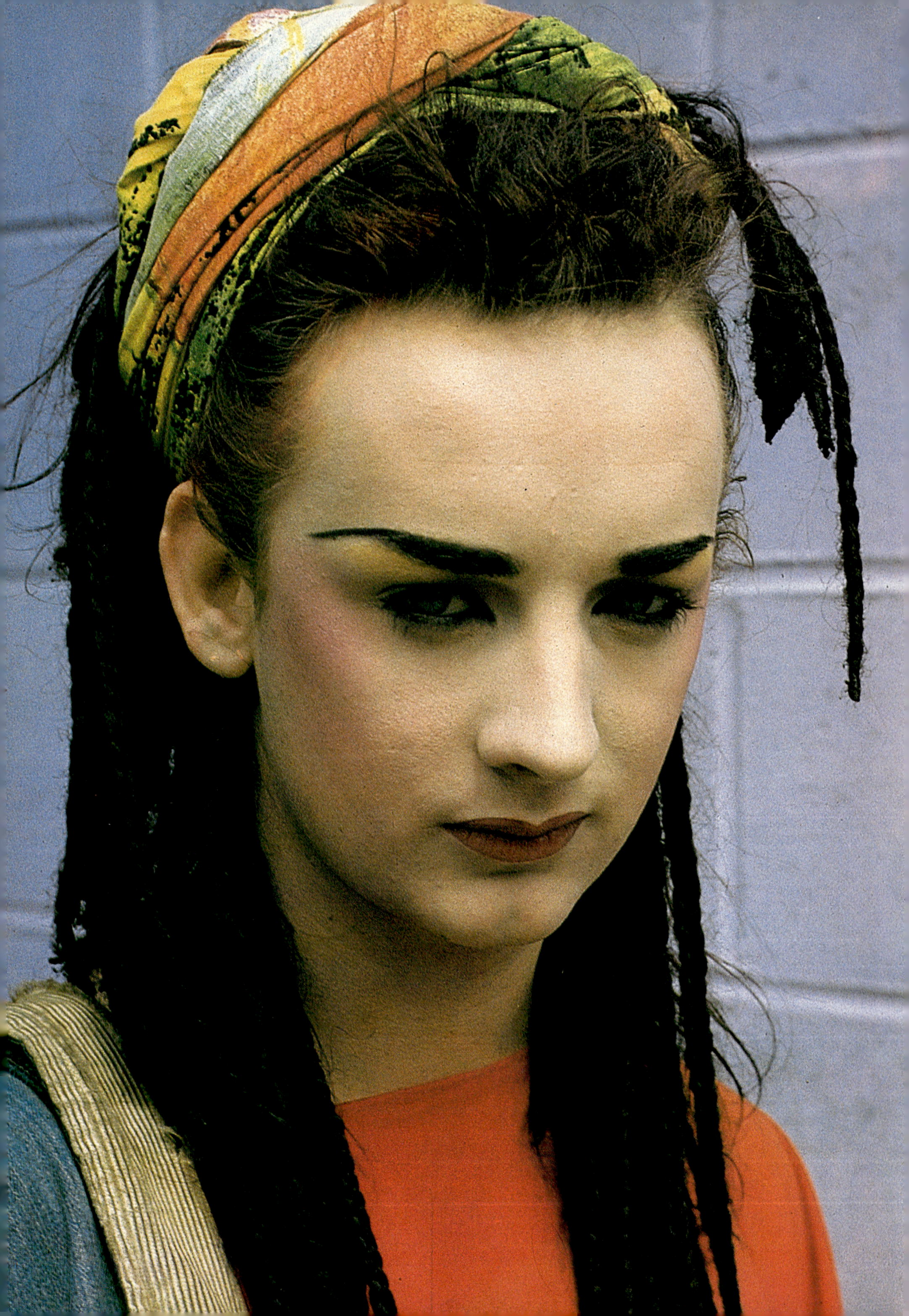

“When I first used make-up I used to do it very badly. But when you get good at it you just want to cover your whole face with it. Of course, dressing up in front of the mirror is one thing, but going out in the street and facing the public is another.”

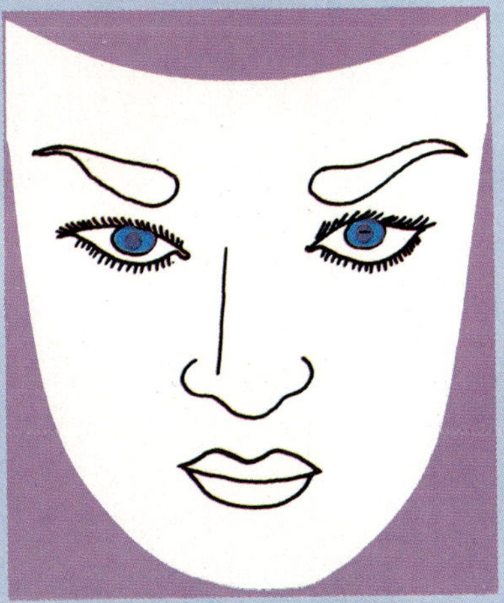

Foundation/Powder: This gentler, coquettish look is achieved by applying a coat of pale pink foundation all over the face to emphasize eyes and mouth. This tends to give a matt finish so brush on some talc for a light sheen. *See page 41.*

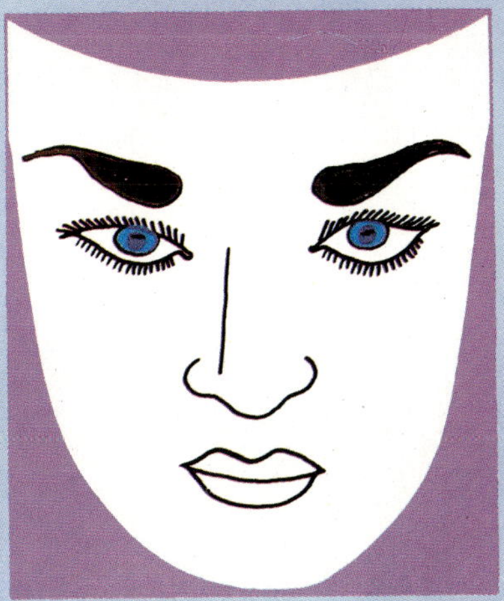

Eyebrows: The brows here are wide, going considerably beyond the natural line. Most people prefer pencils to powder or eye-liner, but the choice is up to you – whichever you select, build up slowly to the correct shape. For methods of application, *see page 41.*

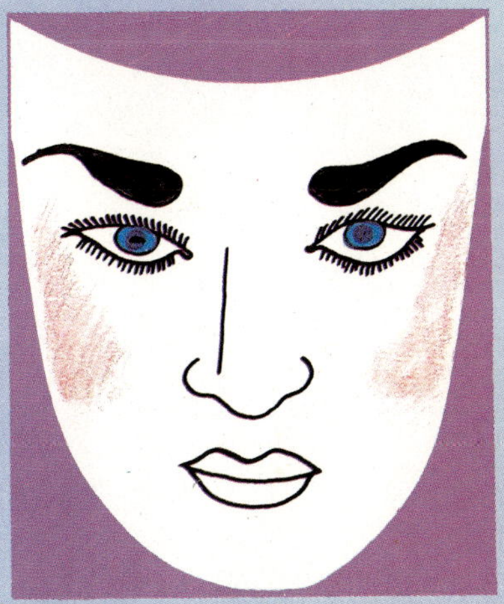

Blusher: Using a dark pink blusher and big brush, apply blush to upper cheek very close to outer corner of eye. Blend down cheekbone softly.

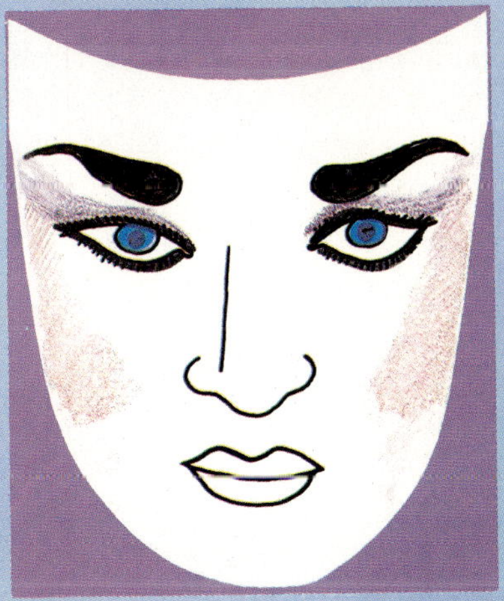

Eyes 1: Outline eye in black pencil or black eye-liner keeping the line close to the lashes. Emphasize inner corner of the eye with same liner or pencil.

Next take burgundy shadow and draw in socket line, quite strong at inner corner fading into socket area.

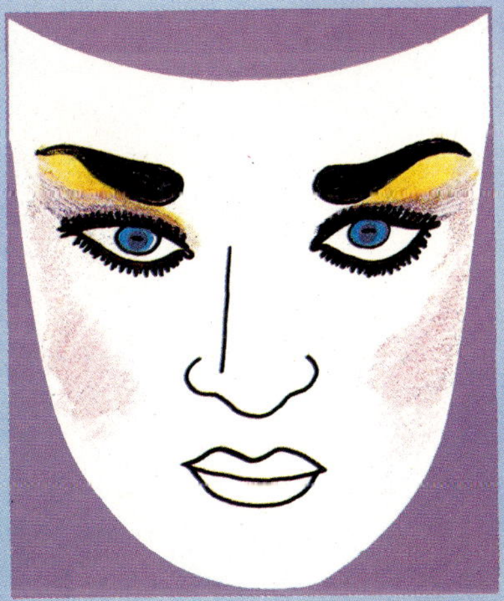

Eyes 2: Using yellow shadow fill in brow bone area and lid taking the color very softly under the eyes. Blend with burgundy in socket.

The lashes are softer here needing just one layer of mascara. Don't forget, however, to brush the lashes through once the mascara has dried.

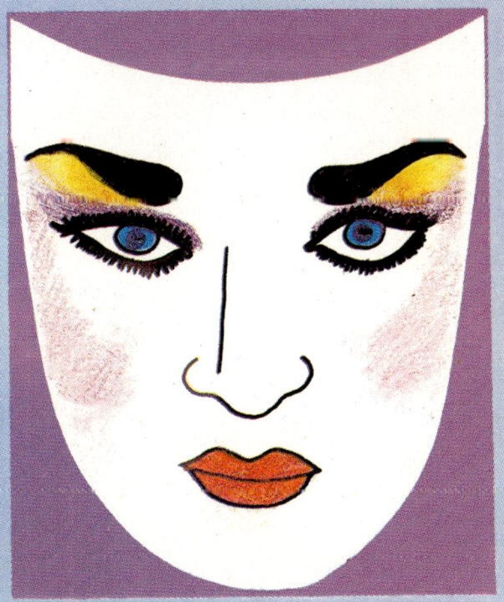

Lips: Using red lipstick and brush, paint in rounded bow-shaped lips. Blot with tissue, powder and re-apply lipstick for longer lasting effect.

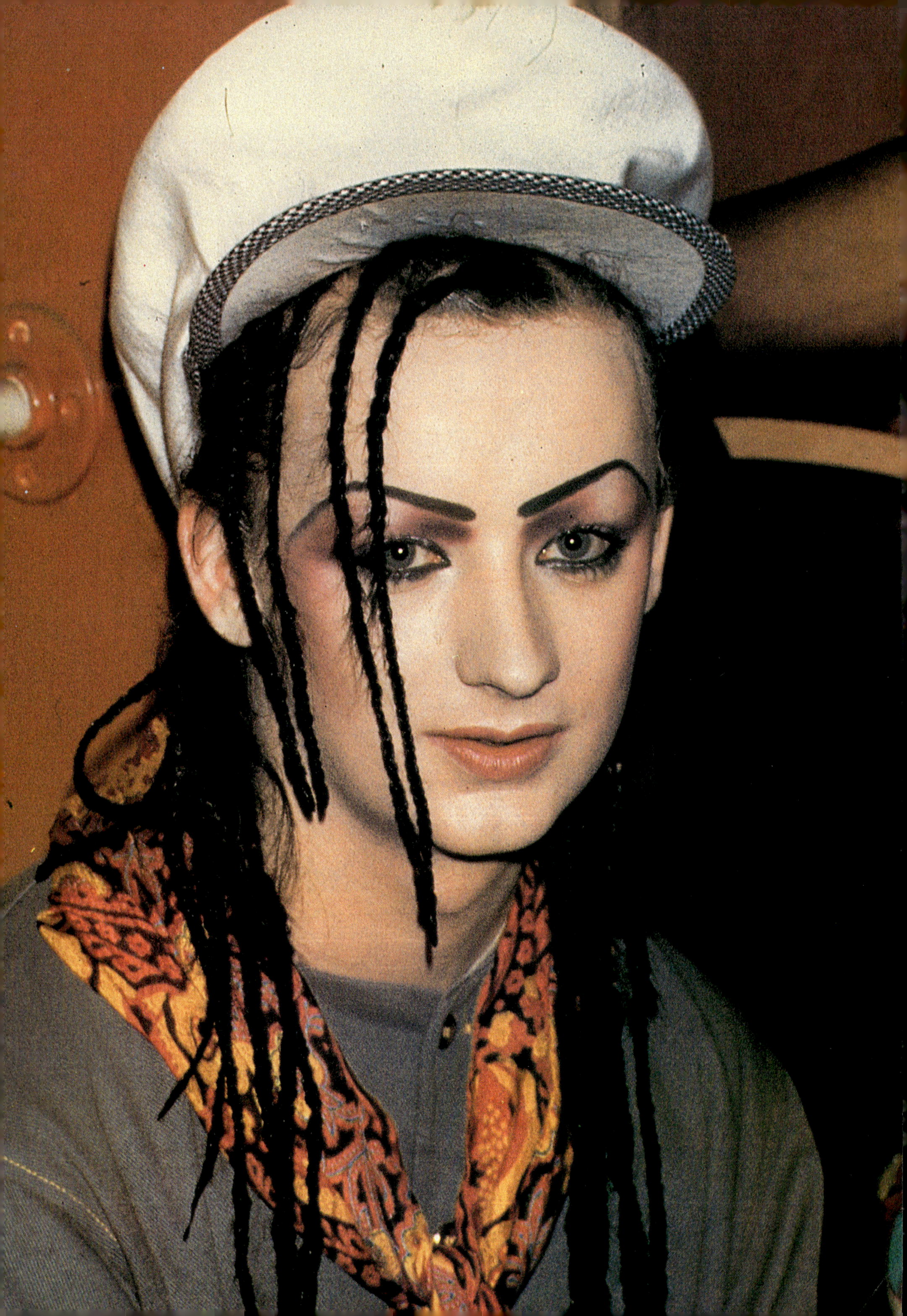

◀ ◀ ◀

Step 1: Wash and condition hair as you would normally and comb through thoroughly while still wet.
Step 2: Divide hair into small square sections all over head, making sure all partings are even. The easiest way to do this is to make two parallel partings, starting over the centre of the forehead and taking them down to the back of the neck. Then with a finger or the pencil end of a comb, divide this 'mohawk streak' into seven or eight even sections. Repeat the process from front to back on both sides of head.
Step 3: Take strands of false nylon hair and plait tightly into own hair, starting at centre front. Make sure as you do this that you plait the hair in the direction you want the plait to fall.
Step 4: To secure plait you can use cotton thread or small rubber bands to tie ends.
Step 5: Repeat this process of plaiting hair and securing the ends all over the head. You may wish to enlist the help of a friend to make it easier.
Step 6: Keep the plaits in for as long as you like. When you want to wash hair, shampoo and condition, concentrating on the scalp.

▶ ▶ ▶

Step 1: Apply mousse or gel to wet hair and toss hair forwards, drying it upside down with hair dryer. You will be surprized by how much thicker your hair will seem as a result of this simple process.
Step 2: Divide hair into sections at the back and sides of head, following the method used earlier for plaiting, only starting at the back.
Step 3: Weave long strands of nylon hair into your own by plaiting for about one inch and securing with cotton thread.
Step 4: You may wish to add brightly colored strands of wool or ribbon or fabric to jazz it up even more.
Step 5: Back-comb your own hair and brush out over false hair to cover roots where false hair has been applied.
Step 6: Tie hair accessories chosen for the occasion around head. These can be used to lift false hair and to give extra volume.

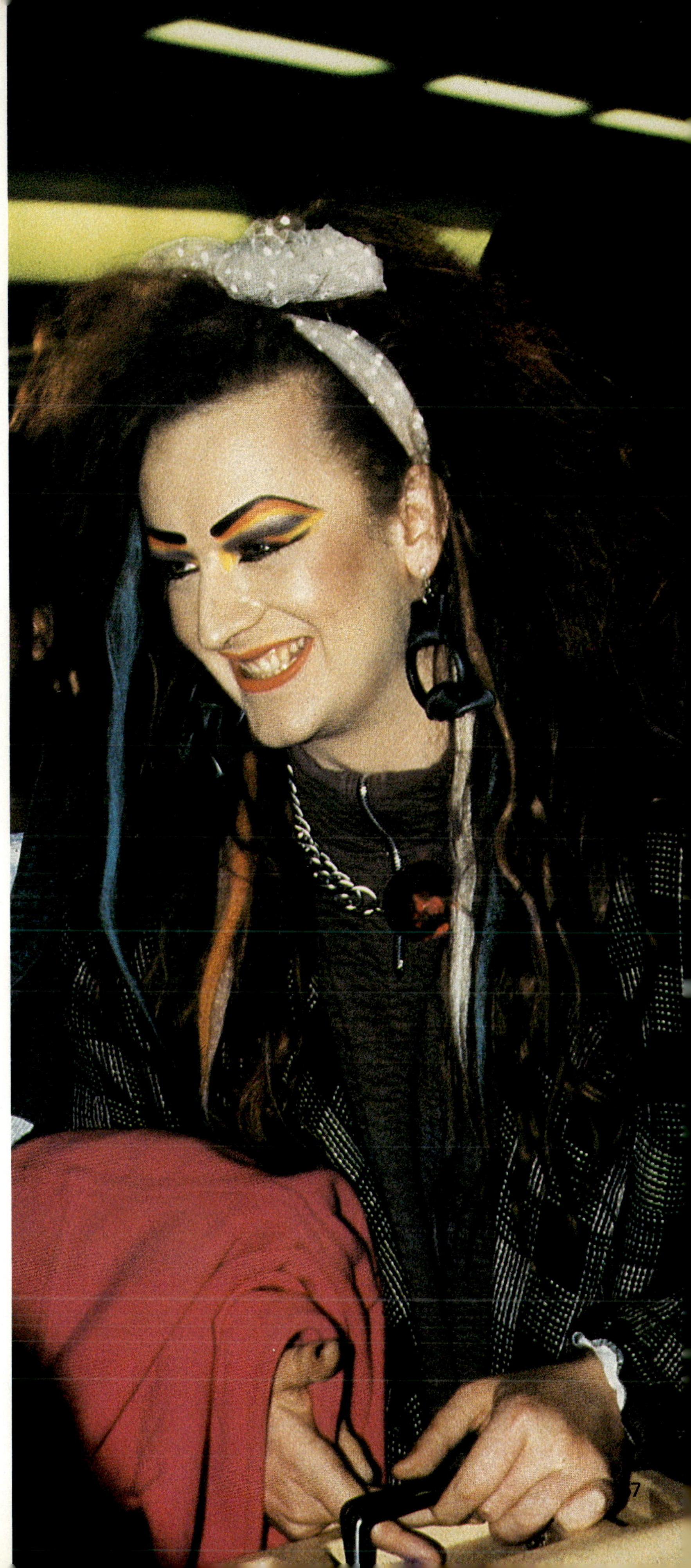

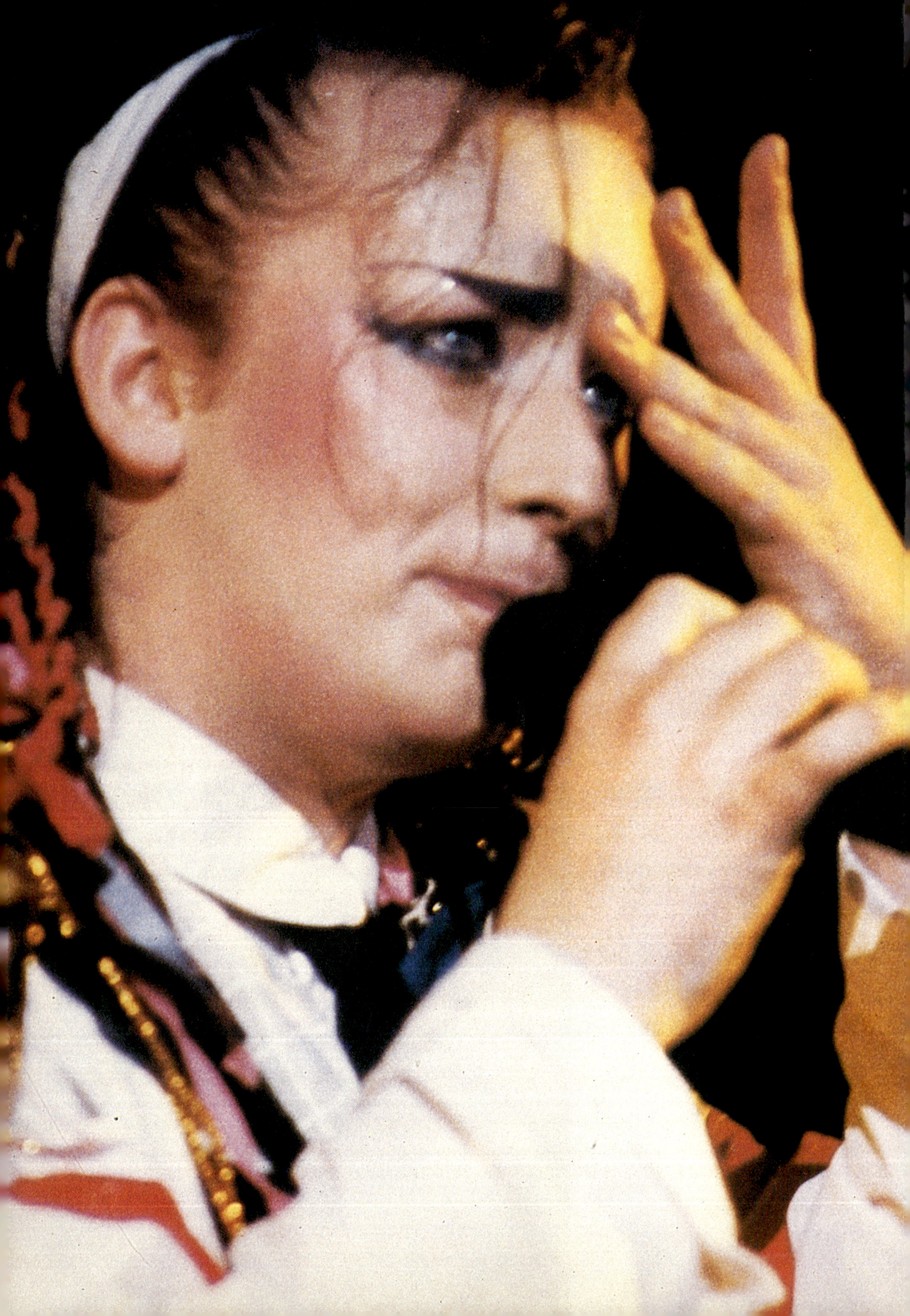

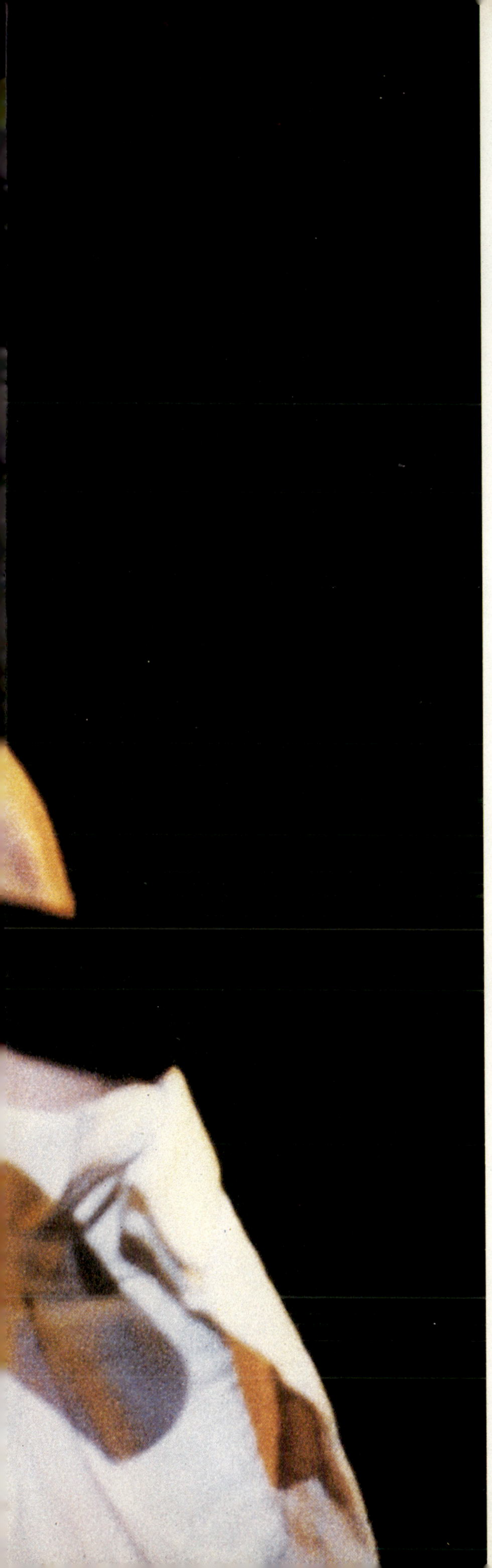

“I think the whole idea of trying to be like everyone else is completely insane.”

“I decided to look more outrageous than everyone else with the make-up and the dresses – but I didn't want to look really awful and just slop the stuff on and look like an idiot. I wanted to look classy. I wanted to look pretty – not grotesque.”

“I've always been like I am, even at school. People think because you dress up you're just adding flames to the fire. That's not true. I'm exactly the same with or without make-up. Except that people are a bit more edgy with me when I am wearing make-up.”

“You have to have a lot of self confidence and you have to be yourself. Otherwise you look like a ham. I don't think I ever looked like a ham. I always thought I looked better than anyone else and that's what kept me going.”

“People say Boy George wears a dress but I'm not a drag queen. I don't wear dresses. My clothes are a male/female mix.”

“You get kids coming to the gigs and they've got loads of make-up on and their hair in wool. They're trying to look like us. But I think when you've got people doing it because they're into it and they're enjoying themselves, that's great.”

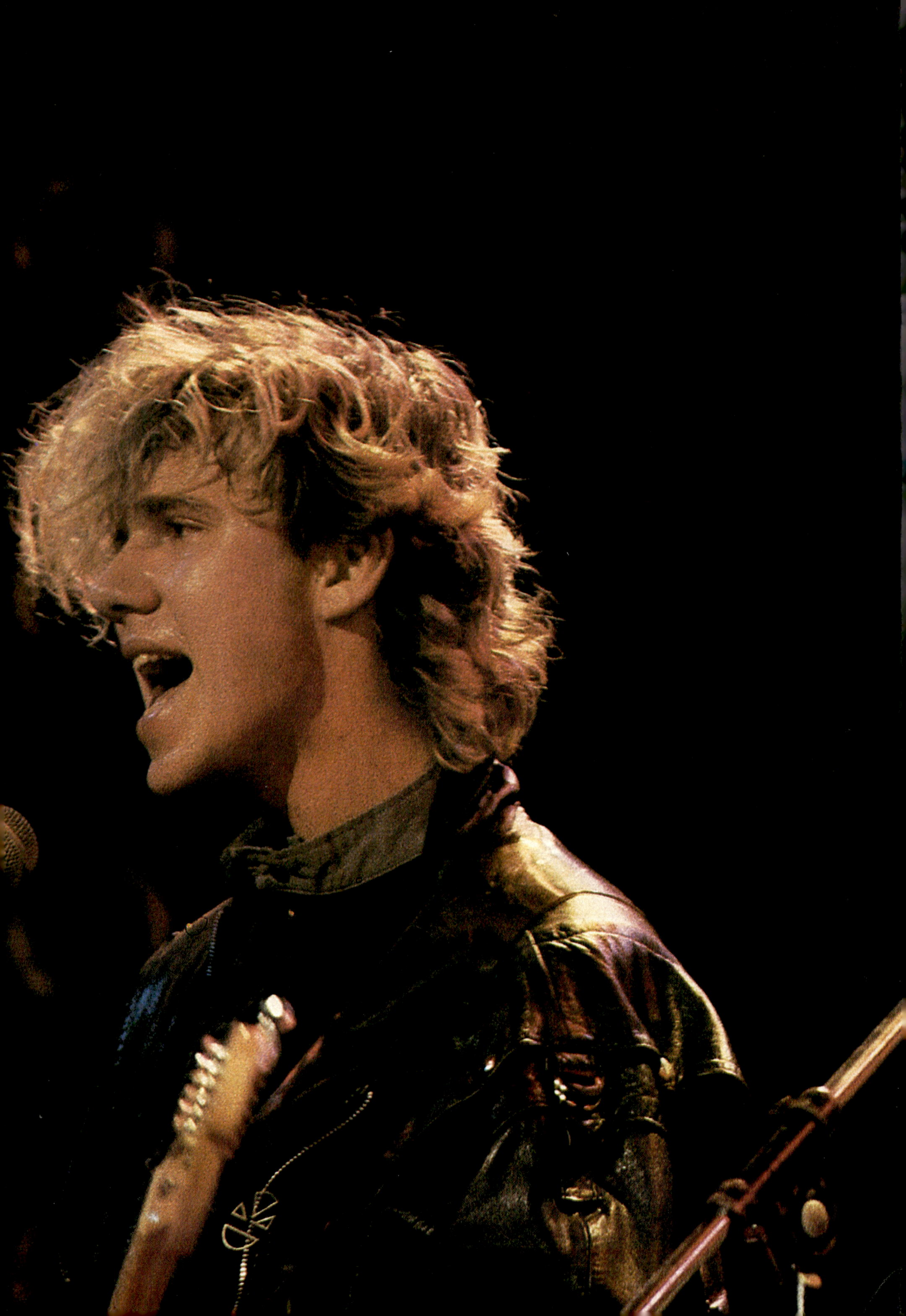

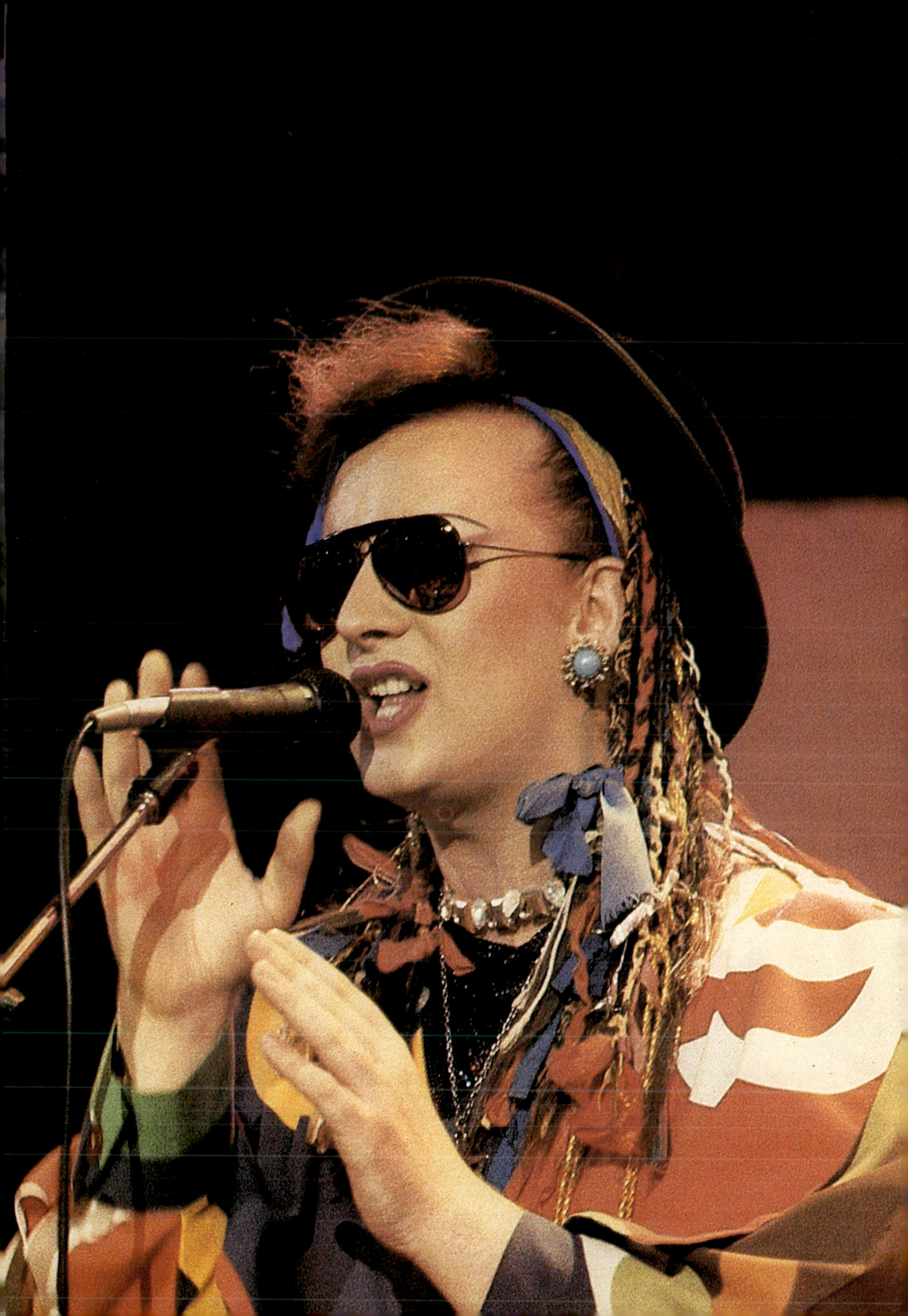

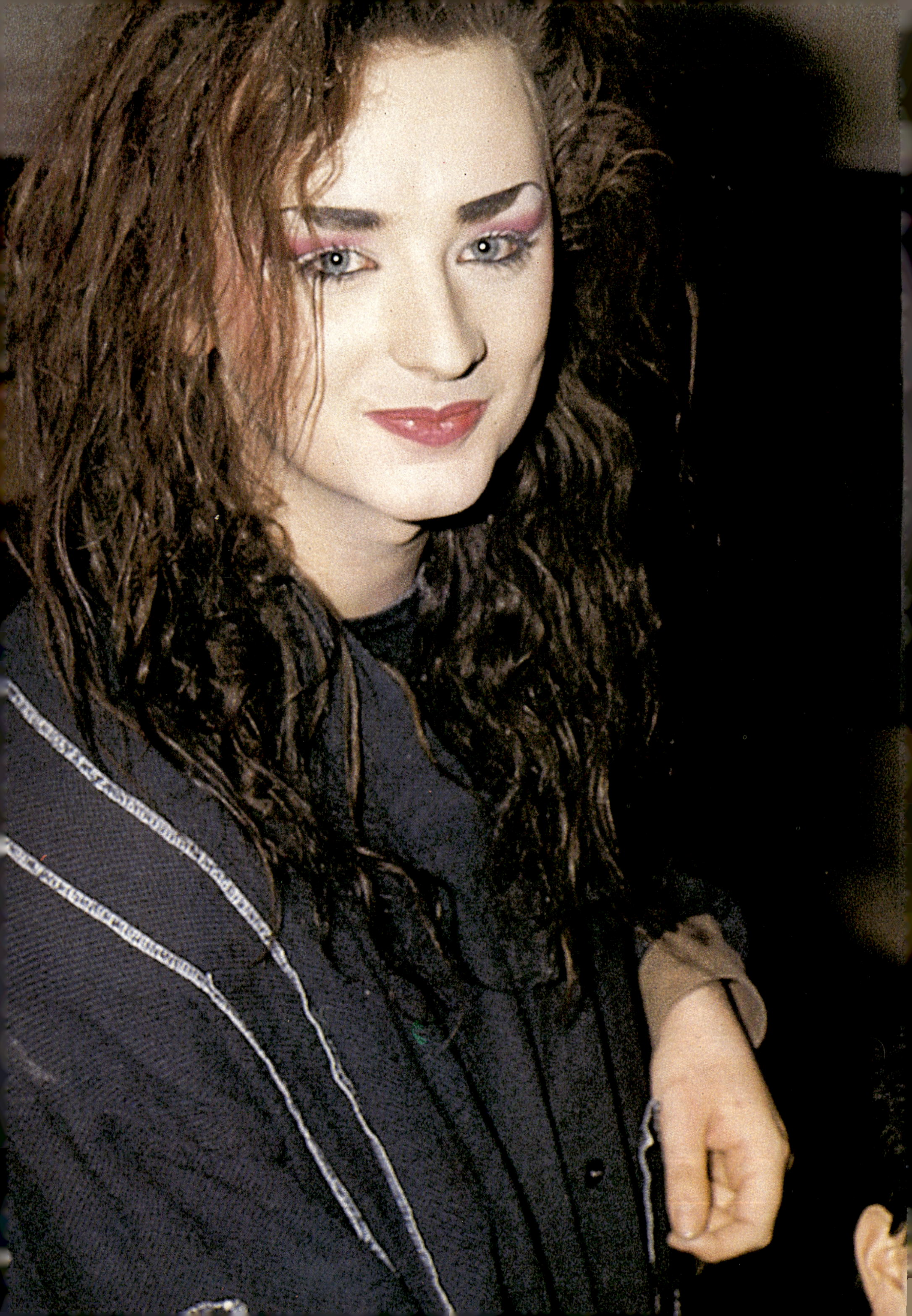

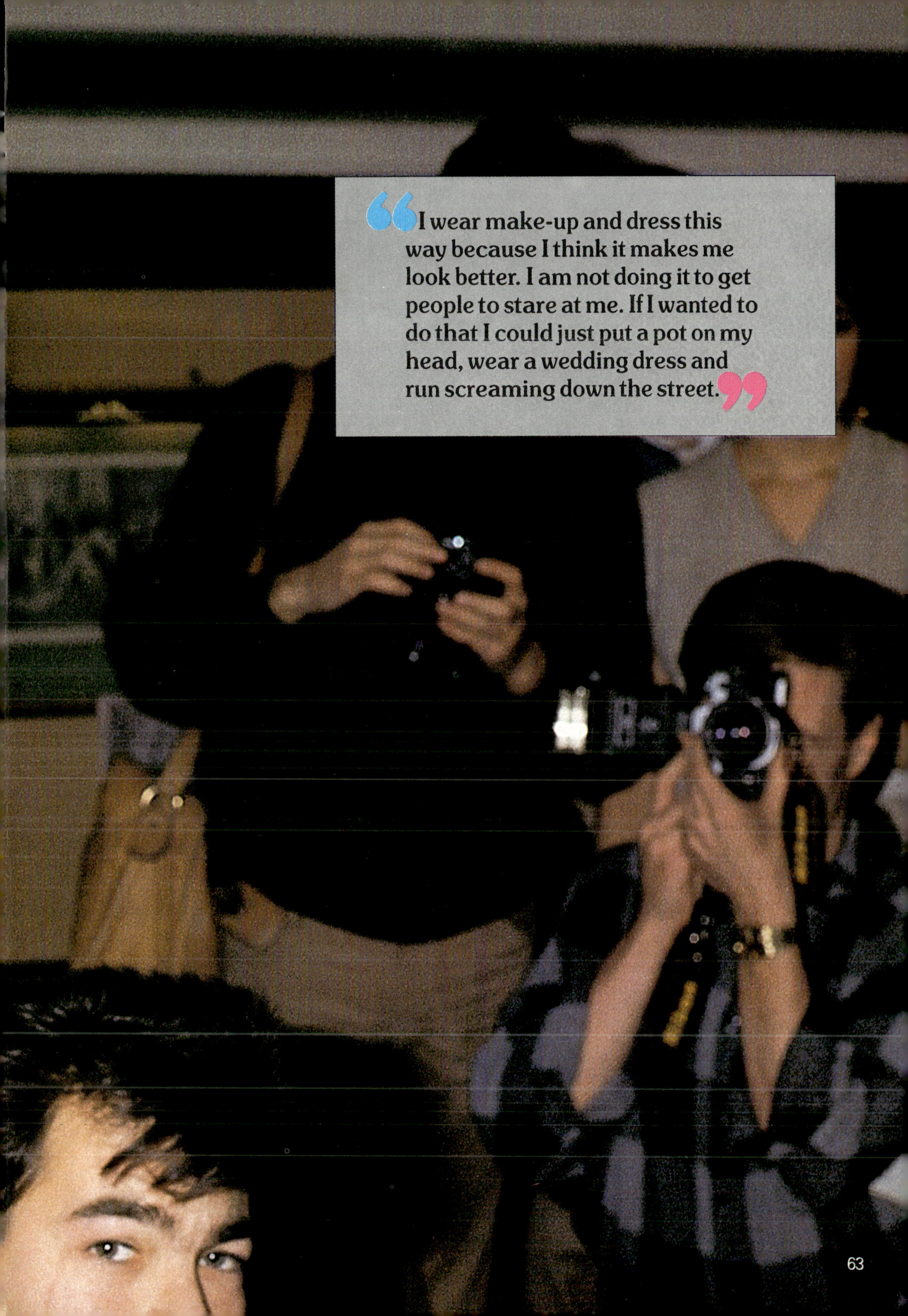

"I wear make-up and dress this way because I think it makes me look better. I am not doing it to get people to stare at me. If I wanted to do that I could just put a pot on my head, wear a wedding dress and run screaming down the street."

Picture Acknowledgements

Andrew Catlin 28, **Colorific!**/Brian Moody/Sunday 40, **London Features International** 1, 3, 6-7, 12, 14, 16, 20, 35, 36-37, 52, 54, 58, 60-61, 62, **Photo Features International Ltd.** 46, **Rex Features** 4-5, 18, 22, 24, 30, 32, 38-39, 44, 50, 56, **Frank Spooner Pictures** 34, **Virgin Records** 42

Multimedia Publications (UK) Limited have endeavoured to observe the legal requirements with regard to the rights of the suppliers of graphic and photographic materials.

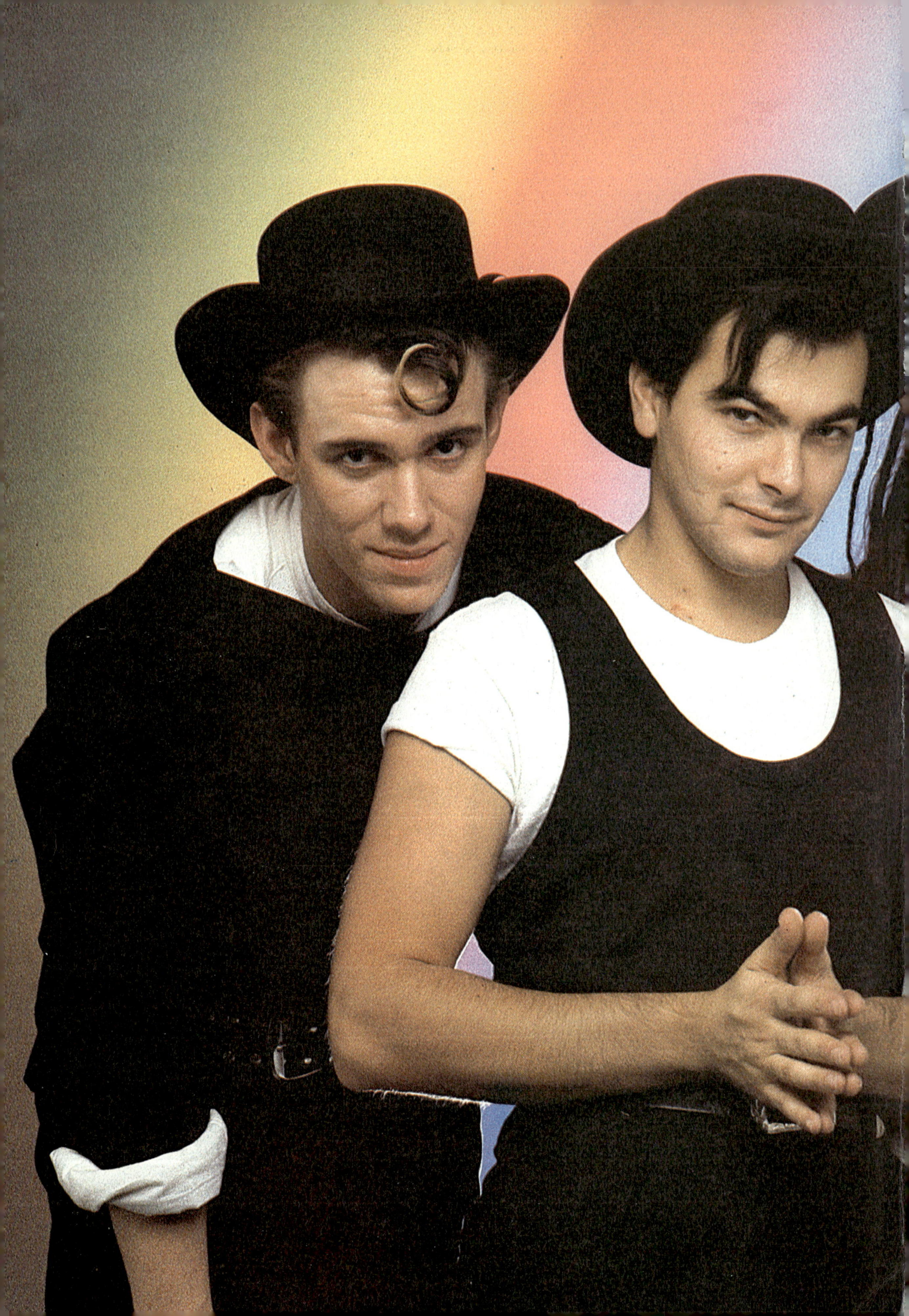